Children
Affected by **HIV/AIDS**

Children
Affected by **HIV/AIDS**

Compassionate Care

Edited by

Phyllis Kilbourn

MARC

800 West Chestnut Avenue, Monrovia, California 91016-3198 USA

10 09 08 07 06 05 04 03 02   4 3 2 1

MARC books are published by World Vision International, 800 West Chestnut Avenue, Monrovia, California 91016–3198, U.S.A.

About the cover:
Uganda AIDS orphans stand next to the front door of their house.

Permissions:
All Scripture quotations, unless otherwise indicated, are from the New Revised Standard Version of the Bible, copyright © 1989 by the Division of Christian Education of the National Council of the Churches of Christ in the USA. Used by permission. All rights reserved.

Poem taken from *Roses in December.* Copyright © 1998 by Marilyn Heavilin. Published by Harvest House Publishers, Eugene, OR 97402. Used by permission.

Poetry and excerpts taken from *Walking with My Lord: A Collection of Poems,* 2nd ed., copyright © 1988 by the Sakuma Family, Montebello, CA. Published by Media Bridge Technologies. Used by permission.

Permission to adapt and use material from Camp Heartland website granted by Neil Willenson, Founder and President of Camp Heartland.

The poem "A Heritage of Death" by Patricia Morgan is from the book *Tell Me Again: The Cry of the Children,* published by Destiny Image Publishers, copyright © 1996. Used by permission of the author.

Editor in Chief: Edna Valdez. Senior editor: Rebecca Russell. Copy editing and typesetting: Joan Weber Laflamme/jml ediset. Cover design: Karen Newe/3 Graces Art & Design. Cover photo: David Ward/World Vision.

This book is printed on acid-free, recycled paper.

Library of Congress Cataloging-in-Publication Data

Children affected by HIV/AIDS : compassionate care / edited by Phyllis Kilbourn.
        p. cm.
Includes bibliographical references.
    ISBN 1-887983-28-7 (alk. paper)
  1. AIDS (Disease) in children. 2. AIDS (Disease) in children—Religious aspects—Christianity. 3. Children of AIDS patients. 4. Children of AIDS patients—Religious aspects—Christianity. I. Kilbourn, Phyllis.
    RJ387.A25 C646 2001
    362.1'98929792—dc21

                                                        2001004750

Contents

CONTENTS

PART IV: STRATEGIES FOR COMPASSIONATE ACTION

PART V: SUSTENANCE FOR CAREGIVERS

PART VI: FIRST-PERSON PERSPECTIVE

Contributing Authors

SNOWDEN ALBRIGHT HOWE is a native North Carolinian and a graduate of the University of North Carolina at Chapel Hill. She received a master's degree in theological studies at Gordon-Conwell Theological Seminary in 1998, with an emphasis in counseling. Currently Howe is preparing for state licensing as a counselor. She is employed by Agape Christian Counseling, Inc.

SUSIE HOWE, an HIV nurse-specialist in hospital and community settings for several years in London, was founder and director of the Bethany Project community-based orphan care program in Zvishavane, Zimbabwe. She is currently director of Scripture Gift Mission International's Pavement Project and is involved in formulating Bible-based resources for the restoration of street children.

PAUL HUDSON is a graduate of Johns Hopkins in Baltimore, Maryland, USA. Experienced in clinical internal medicine, health ministry development and epidemiology, Paul spent several years as a missionary doctor in Ethiopia and Nepal with SIM International. Currently he is serving as SIM International's consultant for health, development and AIDS ministries and contributes articles to several publications.

NANCY HUFF is president and founder of Teach the Children International, an organization that helps establish Christian schools in developing countries and implements programs to teach children to minister. She has written numerous magazine articles on ministry to children at risk and authored two books: *Little Feet with a Big Message*, a how-to book on mobilizing children for outreach, and *Leaving Magnolia*, a book dealing with child abuse.

CONTRIBUTING AUTHORS

PHYLLIS KILBOURN holds the Ph.D. in education from Trinity International University, Deerfield, Illinois. She has served in Liberia and Kenya with WEC International and is currently director of WEC's program for children in crisis, Rainbows of Hope. Kilbourn has traveled in more than 40 countries, researching the needs of children living in difficult circumstances. She has edited or co-edited four other books in this series.

ANN NOONAN is a Licensed Professional Counselor who, in addition to carrying a full caseload, supervises master's level counselors for licensure in North Carolina. Noonan is executive director of Agape Christian Counseling, Inc., in Charlotte, North Carolina, and currently serves as president of the Carolinas Christian Counselors Fellowship. Noonan is also a member of the Charlotte/Mecklenburg Domestic Violence Advisory Board.

MARY REEVES qualified in medicine at Southampton University, England, specializing in pediatrics. A move to South Africa gave Reeves opportunities to witness the many children affected by HIV/AIDS. Working with Healthcare Christian Fellowship International, she is now engaged in training and equipping others globally to care for the emotional and spiritual needs of children with HIV/AIDS.

JANICE SAKUMA, a teacher by profession, is an advocate for children with HIV/AIDS. Losing her daughter to AIDS created within her a deeper calling to minister to children and the hemophilia/AIDS community. She served on the core planning committee to establish The Women's Outreach Network of The National Hemophilia Foundation, known as WONN, and organized the first WONN support group in Southern California for women living with HIV/AIDS. She is an avid speaker and writer, addressing various AIDS issues.

GLEN SLABBER initially worked as an administrator with WEC International in South Africa. Research trips into Zambia and Zimbabwe brought him an awareness of the need for training programs in the field of HIV/AIDS care and education. Slabber has developed a program and manual to train church members in home-based care skills. He is now involved full-time with church member training. He also cooperates with local Bible colleges in preparing student pastors to meet the HIV/AIDS challenge.

DANIEL SWEENEY, an assistant professor in the Graduate Department of Counseling at George Fox University (GFU) in Portland, Oregon, is a licensed therapist, a Registered Play Therapist and Supervisor, and maintains a private practice. He has established a play therapy training program at GFU and is author or co-author of several works on play therapy, including *Play Therapy Interventions with Children's Problems* and *Counseling Children Through the World of Play*, as well as editor of *The Handbook of Group Play Therapy*.

Acknowledgments

Children are like magnets, irresistibly drawing adults into their world. Who hasn't seen a modern-day Pied Piper ambling through a town or a city park? My dad became one of those Pied Pipers whenever he headed to the ice cream parlor on a hot, lazy summer day. He inevitably had a parade of little ones skipping along beside him in anticipation of the treat that was sure to be forthcoming.

That is how it has been in writing this book. Knowing the desperate plight of children affected by HIV/AIDS, compassionate hearts have been drawn together toward a common purpose: preparing a training tool for the children's caregivers who, in turn, will bless the little ones affected by the monster—HIV/AIDS—that has invaded their once carefree world.

The diversity of authorship—practioners, community educators, psychologists, mission strategists, those from the medical profession—and their collective insights and expertise have provided a valuable resource for those attempting to cope with the awesome task of being compassionate caregivers to the millions of children who desperately need help living through the tragedy and brokenness of AIDS.

Special appreciation must be expressed to Janice and Ken Sakuma for allowing the use of their daughter's poems and also for freely sharing their own personal pain, struggles and triumphs as they cared for Stefanie as she suffered from hemophilia related HIV/AIDS.

I join with the children in expressing deepest appreciation for each writer who has joined this journey on behalf of the children and their families. Their gifts of time and expertise are valuable gifts that I do not take for granted. Each writer has many responsibilities and a full workload; writing for this book has been a sacrifice of their time.

Our collective anticipated reward will be witnessing children receiving compassionate care from well-informed caregivers who are aware of their special needs.

Indeed, that will be more than abundant reward for all the efforts poured into this training handbook.

Foreword

Recently I was in South Africa, studying the impact of the growing pandemic of HIV/AIDS. As I stood in the back of the church talking with a doctor friend, he mentioned that three out of five of the young mothers having babies in South Africa today are HIV positive. I was shocked. "Yes," he repeated, "and not only in the black and colored communities—it is true throughout our country."

The next afternoon I was having tea with a pastor friend. I mentioned what the doctor had told me the night before and asked if it was consistent with what he was seeing. "AIDS is the silent disease," the pastor told me. "No one will talk about it, no one will admit it, but I am holding five funerals a week in my church."

The International Conference on AIDS in Africa, held in September 1999, was sponsored by the United Nations and the World Health Organization. Ministers of health from around the world, the heads of African states and 6,000 other concerned persons participated. SIM (Society for International Ministries) and our related churches sent a team of 25 participants. Our delegates, who came from Asia, South America, East Africa, West Africa and South Africa, were saddened at what they heard. "No cure exists," they were told. "Nothing the governments have tried worked, but they don't know what else to do. . . . Just keep on doing the same old things, only faster."

After that conference our representatives met for an additional week. They realized that the experts did not have the answers. In fact, they heard them asking the churches for help. It appears the experts are admitting that the answers are not medical.

Phyllis Kilbourn has correctly identified AIDS as one of the most significant factors affecting the world's children and one of the greatest challenges confronting the church and missions. The number of

HIV-positive adults is doubling every three years. Business people would love to see their businesses grow that fast, but this is not a happy growth curve. More than 20 percent of the adults in Africa are HIV positive at the beginning of this new millennium. If the current rate of growth continues, fully one-half of the adults of Africa will be dead or dying of AIDS within 10 years. Statistics on other continents are not yet as alarming, but current trends indicate that they are heading in the same direction.

But God has not given us a spirit of despair. As our team gathered that week, its members tried to look at the situation from God's perspective. God is aware of the exponential growth in the number of people who are dying and children who are left as orphans. The question for us is what God wants us to do as we walk into the world of tomorrow. We believe we can serve the Lord and help God's church become holy, loving and caring by means of AIDS-related ministries. This book spells out countless opportunities for such involvement.

Yes, we look to the Lord to help us understand how to serve God through compassionate care for children who are growing up in a world in the grip of AIDS. May the Lord give us wisdom to love and help the little ones know God's love.

—ELDON J. HOWARD
SIM DEPUTY GENERAL DIRECTOR

Introduction

The plight of children affected by HIV/AIDS is one of the greatest challenges facing the church and missions today and into the next decade. Think about the AIDS orphan situation. As members of Christ's body, we must be on the cutting edge of response to the overwhelming needs of those affected by the AIDS pandemic. The lives of entire families are affected. For every child directly infected, many more are deeply affected by loss of parents, siblings, other crucial caregivers and the stabilizing factors in their lives.

Knowledge about AIDS and its impact on children is the first step to developing a compassionate ministry. Section I in this book brings awareness and global perspective to the AIDS pandemic. In the light of overwhelming need, we may be tempted to think there is little we can do to offer an effective response. While it is true we may not be able to do much medically, there is a lot we can do through compassionate care. This section starts us on the pathway to compassionate care by describing the "required dress" for compassionate caregiving.

Along with an awareness of the overwhelming need, there must be a Bible-based response. Section II first describes how a mother responded with compassionate care to her child affected by HIV. Then it focuses on how we, members of the body of Christ, are mandated to respond biblically through the church and in missions. Theological foundations for church and mission involvement are clearly laid out along with several practical ways to respond.

Section III covers vital issues surrounding compassionate care: the role of touch and play, longing for relationships, coping with bereavement and loss, and providing spiritual nurture. All are compassionate measures that strike deep chords of needs from

1

children affected by HIV/AIDS, needs, however, that are seldom addressed.

Section IV provides principles for building successful intervention plans to meet the multifaceted needs of those infected and/or affected by AIDS. Possibilities for orphan care, one of the most critical needs, and the "how to's" of providing community education, so vital to prevention, are explored.

Section V addresses caregivers' issues that are vital in keeping the compassion of caregivers vibrant and alive. Being properly prepared can facilitate an effective AIDS ministry. A focus in this section is training for caregivers. Education and training take various forms, but they are indispensable. Learning about AIDS care goes beyond learning about the disease and the physical implications. Caregivers must also learn about the psychosocial aspects of the disease. The social, emotional and economic impact, along with multiple losses, can be as destructive to those affected by HIV/AIDS as the physical losses.

The last section is a tribute to those who are compassionately caring for children with AIDS and encouragement that the long, arduous days invested in children suffering with AIDS are not in vain. As you walk with Stefanie on her courageous journey, you immediately sense that this journey was made possible only through compassionate care. Caregivers can make a difference in the lives of those suffering from HIV/AIDS. However, we, like Stefanie, may need to take courageous steps of faith to become compassionate caregivers to a world affected by the invasion of HIV/AIDS.

PART I

Introduction

1

A Global Window on the HIV/AIDS Crisis

Phyllis Kilbourn

Since the AIDS pandemic was ignited in the late 1970s, the virus has spread like wildfire to every corner of the globe, touching the lives of the youngest to the oldest. An estimated 36.1 million children and adults were living with AIDS at the start of this century. In Africa, 17 million have died since the intrusion of AIDS, including more than 3.7 million children; an additional 12 million children were orphaned.[1] A young AIDS sufferer, assigned to Crib No. 17 in a busy hospital ward, paints the tragic backdrop for all AIDS sufferers:

In Crib No. 17 of the spartan but crowded children's ward at the Church Of Scotland Hospital in KwaZulu-Natal, a tiny, staring child lies dying. She is three and has hardly known a day of good health. Now her skin wrinkles around her body like an oversize suit, and her twig-size bones can barely hold her vertical as nurses search for a vein to take blood. In the frail arms hooked up to transfusion tubes, her veins have collapsed. The nurses palpate a thread-like vessel on the child's forehead. She mews like a wounded animal as one tightens a rubber band around her head to raise the vein. Tears pour unnoticed from her mother's eyes as she watches the needle tap-tap at her daughter's temple. Each time the whimpering child lifts a wan hand to brush away the pain, her mother gently lowers it. Drop by drop, the nurses manage to collect 1 cc of blood in five minutes.[2]

Although we occasionally catch glimpses of the catastrophic destruction this virus has spawned, the immensity and gravity of the AIDS pandemic is seldom fully grasped; AIDS remains largely a silent tragedy. No longer considered only a disease of drug users and homosexuals, the AIDS epidemic runs rampant, showing no respect for age, gender, race, or culture. In fact, AIDS also breaks the normal rules of dying, striking predominantly the young, not the old.

For every child infected with HIV, many more are deeply affected by loss of parents, siblings, other crucial caregivers and all the stabilizing factors that may spell the difference between a healthy childhood and a disaster. This chapter provides a global overview of the crisis, examines causes for the epidemic and highlights its tremendous impact on children.

GLOBAL OVERVIEW OF THE SPREAD OF HIV/AIDS

The American Association for World Health[3] states that 95 percent of all HIV-infected people live in developing regions of the world where social, economic, cultural and political conditions contribute to the spread of the virus. They also state that if the spread of HIV is not contained, AIDS may increase infant mortality by as much as 75 percent and mortality in children under five by more than 100 percent by the year 2010 in regions most affected by the disease. Statistics become outdated daily; however, the constantly rising figures denotes the rapid speed with which AIDS is fanning out across the globe.[4]

Every continent, every country, every city has its own tragic stories to narrate. The following brief overview shows the extent to which this global tragedy is destroying our children's future; it also highlights the urgent need for an immediate and compassionate response.

Africa

The pandemic of AIDS has changed Africa forever. A 1999 report from the United Nations[5] stated that AIDS, not war, has turned Africa into a "killing field" that would wipe out enough adults to create 13 million orphans in the following eighteen months. Within the African continent, sub-Saharan Africa is still

6

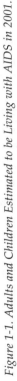

Figure 1-1. Adults and Children Estimated to be Living with AIDS in 2001.

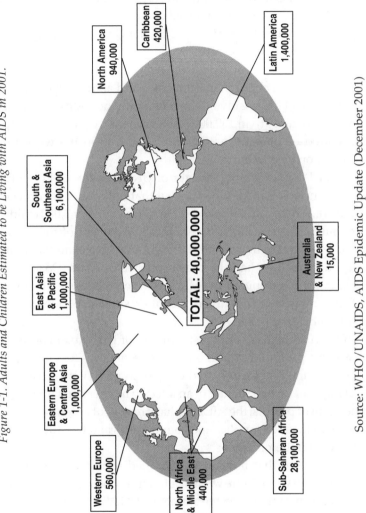

North America
940,000

Caribbean
420,000

Latin America
1,400,000

South &
Southeast Asia
6,100,000

East Asia
& Pacific
1,000,000

Eastern Europe
& Central Asia
1,000,000

Western Europe
560,000

North Africa
& Middle East
440,000

Sub-Saharan Africa
28,100,000

Australia
& New Zealand
15,000

TOTAL : 40,000,000

Source: WHO/UNAIDS, AIDS Epidemic Update (December 2001)

the global epicenter for HIV/AIDS, with over two-thirds of the world's HIV-positive people living in this region. Over 25 million sub-Saharan Africans are estimated to be living with HIV or AIDS. Almost 12 million have died in this region due to AIDS-related illnesses. AIDS also has cut the average predicted life span from 64 to 47 in the nine worst affected countries in Africa.[6]

Zimbabwe has been described by the United Nations as having the worst AIDS problem in the world. The United Nations also states that in the next decade AIDS will orphan approximately 45 percent of all children in Zimbabwe and about half of the children will be HIV positive. In just one province, Masvingo, there are already more than 100,000 AIDS orphans. Agricultural output decreased 62 percent in 1999 due to a drop in the work force brought on by death from AIDS.[7]

Peter Picot, executive director of UNAIDS, the UN organization set up to fight AIDS, points out that millions of African children are at risk from the disease. He states that over 2,000 children are infected every day.[8] An estimated 87 percent of the world's children who are living with HIV live in Africa. And 1.7 million Ugandan children have become orphaned due to AIDS since the beginning of the epidemic.[9] AIDS also is on the rise in other parts of Africa where, if not curbed, it could result in a pandemic similar to sub-Saharan Africa.

For Africa, AIDS is not just a matter of individual concern. It has had a profound impact on and consequences for entire families. An infant or young child diagnosed as HIV positive is frequently the son or daughter of an infected mother and father. Upon the death of parents, the AIDS orphans represent a significant challenge to extended families and communities and face future hardship within their societies.

The groups that have been identified as most susceptible to acquiring HIV/AIDS are women, girls and adolescents. The United Nations has stated that the number of HIV-positive women in Africa has surpassed infected men for the first time.[10] Sexual practices, cultural norms and sometimes unarticulated social expectations all contribute to the high-risk behaviors that make these groups vulnerable. AIDS kills children more rapidly in Africa, partly because of the less developed health-care systems. Many basic antibiotics are unavailable. Children are often weakened by poor nutrition. Typical childhood diseases such as diarrhea and measles often kill children with HIV.

African society, with its strong sense of family, has always provided an expansive network of family members for those who have lost their parents. Today there is a growing number of so-called AIDS orphans—children who have lost their parents and extended family members to AIDS. Statistics show that millions more parents are carriers of the HIV virus that leads to AIDS, indicating millions more children will be orphaned in the next few years. In fact, the United Nations has warned that Africa is in danger of becoming a continent of orphans unless swift action is taken to control the spread of the deadly virus.

North Africa and the Middle East

Less is known about the HIV/AIDS epidemic in North Africa and the Middle East than in other parts of the world. The generally conservative social and political attitudes and traditions in many of the countries in these regions present challenges to HIV/AIDS awareness and prevention efforts among their populations. In 1998, 10,000 new cases of HIV infections were reported; a total of 210,000 people are thought to be living with HIV in this region.[11]

Europe

Many countries in Eastern Europe have reported dramatic growth in HIV infection rates since the early 1990s: 700,000 people were living with HIV at the start of 2000, compared to 420,000 in 1999. In the Federation of Russia there were 130,000 who were AIDS infected in 1999, with an expected rise to 300,000 by 2000; four of every five newly diagnosed infections reported were caused by drugs taken by injection. There were 30,000 new cases of HIV/AIDS reported in 1998. Today there may be nearly four times as many infections in the Ukraine alone as there were in the entire Eastern European region just three years ago.[12]

Asia and the Pacific

In 1998 an estimated 7 million people lived with HIV/AIDS in Asia and the Pacific region—just 1 in 5 of the world's total. By the end of the year 2000 that number was expected to have grown to 1 in 4. The high rates of infection and the rampant spread of HIV in Asia are attributed primarily to sharing needles for drug use and to the commercial sex industry.

India has over 4 million people living with HIV, the largest number of HIV-infected people in any country of the world. In Cambodia 200 people are being infected with HIV every day; by the end of the year 2000, the death rate from AIDS had already produced 43,000 new orphans.[13] In China over 400,000 people were estimated to be living with HIV/AIDS in 1997. The number of HIV-infected people in South and Southeast Asia now exceeds the total number of infected people in the entire industrialized world.

Latin America and the Caribbean

In Latin America and the Caribbean an estimated 1.7 million adults and children were living with HIV by the end of 1998. In this region HIV/AIDS has taken its greatest toll among homosexual men and drug users. However, rising infection rates in women, and, consequently in infants, show that heterosexual transmission is becoming prominent. Traditional mores and attitudes can lead to double standards that encourage men to have many sexual partners. Cultural expectations of female submissiveness and male dominance in sexual relations result in more women being placed at a risk of infection. In addition, the HIV epidemic is shifting to younger populations; the number of young people in this region (ages 15–24) in 1998 who were infected with HIV was over 65,000. In Mexico between 3 percent and 11 percent of injection drug users are HIV infected; in Argentina and Brazil the percentage may be close to 50 percent.

North America

For the United States HIV is the most critical and devastating epidemic in recent history. HIV infection and the clinical complications that result are placing a heavy strain on medical and social services. The Centers for Disease Control and Prevention (CDC)[14] reports the following facts:

- AIDS is the second leading cause of death among adults ages 25–44.
- The total number of HIV-infected persons in the United States is estimated to be between 650,000 and 900,000, and approximately 40,000 people are infected each year.
- Approximately 1 in 300 Americans is HIV-positive: 1 in 160 males, and 1 in 1,000 females.
- Although racial and ethnic minorities account for only 25 percent of the US population, they account for over 50 percent of all AIDS cases.
- More than 410,000 Americans have died of AIDS.

In Canada a cumulative total of 17,165 AIDS cases were diagnosed up to June 30, 2000; 197 were children under 15 years of age. There has been a steady increase in HIV attributable to heterosexual contact and, in contrast, a decrease in those attributable to homosexual contacts. The proportion of HIV-positive test reports among adult women remains at about 20 percent each year.[15]

Although the toll is highest in North America in drug-ridden ghettos, the spread of HIV/AIDS is not just a big-city phenomenon. Rural areas are experiencing a rise in drug usage. Often infected mothers leave large cities and return to the places where they grew up so extended family members can take in their children. Many are simply returning home to die.

As new infections continue to occur and new drug therapies keep people with HIV alive longer, the proportion of the population living with HIV has grown in these regions. Correspondingly, the number of AIDS-related deaths has declined. The shift has caused greater demands for care and presented new prevention challenges.

CAUSES FOR CONTRACTING HIV/AIDS
There are many factors promoting the rapid spread of HIV/AIDS, including sexual promiscuity, poverty, discrimination, drug use, inadequate health or social services, rapid urbanization and a migrant labor force. Many issues also arise from sexual abuse and prostitution, injection drug use and blood transfusion, all which have created environments promoting the spread of the virus.

As caregivers, we need to examine the underlying causes for this spread if we are to plan effective prevention programs—our first line of attack against the extensive spreading of this deadly virus. The following sections highlight some of the major underlying causes for the spread of HIV.

Maternal AIDS

Women of childbearing age now make up an ever-increasing proportion of people with HIV worldwide. By January 1, 1996, 3.2 million children had been infected with HIV through mother-to-child transmission. Of this number, 2.35 million have developed AIDS and 2.29 million have died of AIDS.[16]

The virus can cross the placenta and infect the fetus during pregnancy. The infant can be exposed by contact with the mother's cervical secretions and blood during labor and delivery. Finally, an infant can contract the virus through breast feeding as the baby ingests HIV-infected breast milk.

The determination of whether an infant born to an infected mother has been infected with HIV cannot be made immediately after birth. The blood-screening test that can detect antibodies to HIV does not distinguish between maternal antibodies and antibodies produced by the infant. Maternal antibodies can remain in the infant's system for 9 to 15 months.

A multi-site study in Thailand conducted by the Thai Red Cross Society showed that HIV transmission rates from mother to child ranged from 25 to 42 percent. More than 5,000 children are born each year with HIV. New annual pediatric AIDS cases were predicted to rise from 3,100 in 1993 to 7,000 in 2000.[17]

Poverty

The situation of medical care for children with HIV/AIDS is grim in poverty-stricken nations. These children have little access to basic health care and are unlikely to benefit from the recent advances made in antiviral therapy. Even inexpensive medicines to treat HIV-related illnesses and reduce suffering are not available. In Europe, more than 20 percent of HIV-positive children are still alive at the age of 10. In contrast, a recent study from Zambia

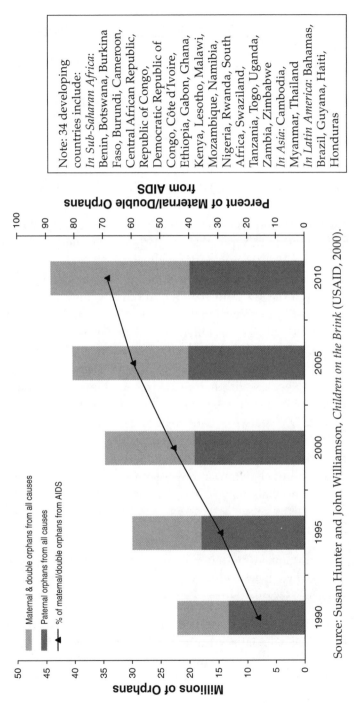

Fig. 1-2. Orphan Estimates for 34 Developing Countries

Source: Susan Hunter and John Williamson, *Children on the Brink* (USAID, 2000).

Note: 34 developing countries include:
In Sub-Saharan Africa: Benin, Botswana, Burkina Faso, Burundi, Cameroon, Central African Republic, Republic of Congo, Democratic Republic of Congo, Côte d'Ivoire, Ethiopia, Gabon, Ghana, Kenya, Lesotho, Malawi, Mozambique, Namibia, Nigeria, Rwanda, South Africa, Swaziland, Tanzania, Togo, Uganda, Zambia, Zimbabwe
In Asia: Cambodia, Myanmar, Thailand
In Latin America: Bahamas, Brazil, Guyana, Haiti, Honduras

showed that nearly 50 percent of HIV-positive children had died by age two.[18]

While poverty is related to a lack of basic needs—food, safe drinking water, shelter and safety—it is often also related to an absence of rights or of access to justice. In many cases there is a chronic lack of hope. Nepal, where 40 percent of the population lives below the subsistence level, is a vivid example of a country with a rapidly rising increase in AIDS cases. The economic factors there have combined with cultural factors to fuel the trade in girls and thus the spread of HIV/AIDS. Factors include women's low status, poverty, migrant workers from high-prevalence countries (like India) and sometimes simply caste prejudice. In 1997, 863 people tested HIV positive; the 1998 figures suggested between 8,000 and 10,000 actual HIV-positive cases.[19]

Kanchi, from Pokhara, and her three young siblings are involved in the sex industry. Due to poverty, they all were forced into prostitution, learning the trade from one another. Before long, one of the siblings was killed by a client. Sex is a taboo subject in Nepal, and this makes AIDS awareness difficult. But the sex trade is a problem of monumental proportions. There are an estimated 100,000 Nepalese girls in Indian brothels alone. Twenty percent of these are under 16 years of age. The number leaving Nepal is around 5,000 per year: over 96 per week, 14 every day.

When an HIV diagnosis occurs in the family, the household often also suffers disproportionately, not only from stigma and isolation but also from impoverishment. A recent study in Thailand found that many parents had lost jobs as a result of AIDS.

Sex Trade

> Prostitution is no future for a child. You just die slowly while giving money to someone else. (13–year-old ex-prostitute with the AIDS virus)

The AIDS epidemic has become both a cause and a consequence of the commercial sex trade of children. When children are orphaned, they become vulnerable to exploitation and abuse. In Asia thousands of orphaned children who have been forced into commercial sex work have become HIV positive. All sexual exploitation and abuse, including that involved in the sale of children, child prostitution, child pornography and early marriages, increase the risk of infection by HIV. Efforts to stop these practices should be part of HIV-prevention concerns.

No one knows how many child sex workers there are in the world, but recent UN figures indicate an estimated 10 million children worldwide are in the sex industry with more than 1 million more entering every year. The HIV/AIDS epidemic has made child sexual abuse and child prostitution more dangerous than ever. The belief that children are less likely to be infected has raised the demand for younger sex workers. Awareness about the scale of child abuse that takes place in or from the home also is slowly growing.

Drugs

Dr. Molly Joel Coye, New Jersey State Commissioner of Health, claims,

> The parallel epidemic that is fueling the HIV epidemic is drug abuse. . . . Despite the war on drugs and recent decreases in casual drug use, drug addiction is increasing and threatens to erode our fragile gains against the transmission of HIV.[20]

Thailand is an example of a nation where the HIV/AIDS epidemic initially gained a foothold in the drug-injecting community. The northeastern states of India are the hot spots of AIDS. In fact, it is the worst affected region of India. The main source of HIV transmission in these states is drug-injecting equipment; the IV drug users constitute the high risk behavior group.[21]

Lack of Education

In terms of reducing vulnerability to infection, children and adolescents are often denied access to HIV education, information, health care and means of prevention—access adults have. This is a violation of the rights of children for nondiscrimination, education and health, as well as a violation of their right to express their own views and to seek, receive and impart information and ideas of all kinds.

IMPACT OF HIV/AIDS ON CHILDREN

More children are contracting HIV than ever before, and there is no sign that the infection rate is slowing. When AIDS decimates a child's family, it results in a relentless onslaught of losses that allows only a brief time to grieve one death before being confronted with another. AIDS' continuing stigma produces silent grievers as children watch helplessly while death sweeps through their families. To prevent loss of work time from families who have five or more funerals to attend weekly, some towns in South Africa conduct funerals only on weekends. Thirty-five fresh children's graves were dug daily in a squatter camp the author visited. People lived in the shadow of death.

Although AIDS is considered the most recognized disease in the world today, the disastrous impact it is having on children has not been given adequate attention. Being the weakest members of society, children are most vulnerable when this catastrophe strikes, swiftly cutting their life expectancy. Estimates quoted in a UNAIDS report indicate that by the year 2,010 AIDS may increase infant mortality by as much as 75 percent and under-five child mortality by more than 100 percent in the most hard-hit countries in the world.[22] This will place AIDS as a major cause of death among children.

Children living in hard-hit communities feel the impact as they lose parents, teachers and caregivers to AIDS, as health systems are stretched beyond their limits and as their families take in other children who have been orphaned by the epidemic. Individual households struck by AIDS often suffer disproportionately from stigma, isolation and impoverishment; the emotional toll on the children is heavier still.

As the number of children orphaned or otherwise affected by AIDS rises, social security systems, already under-funded and overburdened where they exist, are at the breaking point. The impact is most acute on children already facing hardship or neglect: children in institutional care; children in poor neighborhoods or slum areas; refugee children; and even more so for young girls who have unequal opportunities for schooling and employment.

A UNICEF/WHO report describes the impact:

> The effects of the epidemic are starkly obvious from the ba-
> nana plantations going fallow, the houses closed or aban-
> doned, the funeral processions on the roads and the recent
> graves near homes where grandparents care for children
> whose parents have died.[23]

Children, however, do not need to contract AIDS to be profoundly victimized by its impact. Sometimes children's stable
home life is disrupted when their families take in children orphaned through HIV/AIDS. Or they may have to drop out of
school and take care of their parents, struggling to discover ways
to cope with their parents' illness. The stigma and shame associated with AIDS also takes its toil. Society's negative attitudes
deeply affect the children psychologically and emotionally.

When the wage earner in a family is chronically ill, family members also suffer economic deprivation. This leads to poverty, which
means many children have to drop out of school as the parents
become unable to afford the fees. It also means the children are
compelled to work to help support the family. A reversal of roles
occurs, bringing confusion and instability into the lives of the children.

It is inevitable that these children will have to cope with the
loss of one or both parents when they eventually die of AIDS. This
further exacerbates their situation and increases their vulnerability and dependence on society. Watching their parents or other
loved ones die further traumatizes them; the trauma is compounded when they become orphaned.

Young girls are most vulnerable to the impact of HIV/AIDS,
especially children who live in poor neighborhoods or slum areas
and refugee or displaced children. Also at risk are children in in-
stitutions and those who are sexually exploited. According to
UNAIDS, children in developing countries who are infected with
HIV are more likely to die than infected children in industrialized
countries. In Europe 80 percent of HIV-positive children survive
at least until their third year, and more than 20 percent reach the
age of 10 years. But in sub-Saharan Africa, the region currently
most severely affected by AIDS, children have a much poorer survival rate.[24]

INTRODUCTION

Children with HIV/AIDS face many traumas besides their own sickness and impending death. They often first watch their HIV-infected parents slowly grow sicker and eventually experience painful deaths. These events often are accompanied by their families becoming stressed by decreasing resources. Deep traumas stem from those who demonstrate cruel discrimination against children because of their or their parents' sickness. Abandoned or orphaned children, or those who experience undue family pressures, especially from poverty, often wind up living on danger-laden streets.

Discrimination

A traumatic and damaging impact on children is discrimination. As knowledge of their or their parents' illness becomes known, children immediately suffer from society's negative attitudes toward the infected. These attitudes result in discrimination, isolation, stigma and rejection. Other children are not allowed to play with them; they suffer discrimination from classmates and sometimes even teachers at school. Discrimination aimed at parents often includes the loss of their jobs or businesses, forcing children to assume parental responsibilities. Isolated, children often become prisoners in their own home. They are tarred with the same brush as their parents, whether or not they have the virus.

Discrimination can mean that orphans are locked into a vicious circle of deprivation, increased vulnerability to poverty and HIV. "This lady likes mistreating me because my mother is dead," says one Ugandan girl. "She wants me to sleep with men because I stay in her house. She tells me to be good to them and says this is the only way I can continue to live in her house."

Economic hardships

When the wage earner in a family is chronically ill, the family members suffer economic deprivation leading to lack of basic necessities. This soon leads to poverty, which means many children have to drop out of school. It also means the children are compelled to work and earn money to help support the family. This reversal of roles brings confusion and instability into the lives of the children. They lose the security of being cared for.

18

Depression

Society's negative attitudes toward those suffering with HIV/AIDS deeply affect the children psychologically and emotionally. Also, children whose parents are sick with AIDS know they eventually will have to cope with the loss of one or both parents. Studies have shown that HIV-negative children who have mothers with HIV infection are significantly more depressed and are more likely to have problems with attention.[25] Unlike children with the more obvious behaviors of aggression and delinquency, they are less likely to come to the attention of teachers and health professionals.

Moreover, the stigma of AIDS forces many families to keep the cause of death quiet. The surviving children are isolated, living with shame. They don't tell anybody, not even their best friend or teachers. Older children are usually aware that if their parents died from cancer or a car accident, they would receive sympathy, not rejection. Their silence often takes its toll. With no acceptable outlet for their rage or grief, children often cause trouble in school. Boys especially may get in trouble with the police. Some teenagers turn to indiscriminate sex or drug use, almost daring the AIDS virus to do to them what it did to their parents.

ORPHANED BY AIDS

Children who are left when parents die add another complex dimension to the AIDS pandemic. While orphans have been traditionally cared for by their extended family, many communities are becoming saturated with orphans, and families can't afford to take on another child, leaving thousands to fend for themselves. Obo's story paints scenes that vividly describe life as an orphan.

> Obo is 14 and lives in a compound slum in a medium-sized city. Many of the people who live in his community have HIV, the virus that causes AIDS, and many have already died. Obo's mother died of an AIDS-related illness two years ago. After her death his father went away to another town. Obo thinks his father was infected with HIV as well.
>
> Obo now lives with his uncle and works on the streets every day selling food. He would like to be a taxi driver in the future. He also has been trying to save money and to learn to read and write.

> Obo and some of his friends use hashish occasionally. Pills
> . . . have recently become available to the children who work
> on the streets. Obo has tried them once or twice. . . . His uncle
> is worried about him and has talked to him about his con-
> cerns. He wants Obo to have a better future, but he has no
> money to offer him.[26]

Orphans like Obo must learn to fend for themselves in an environment that holds no glimmer of hope for their future. The trauma
orphans suffer from losing parents, and often their homes as well,
is compounded by the struggle simply to survive. Most orphans
drop out of school, suffer malnutrition, receive little if any medical care, and have emotional problems due to unresolved grief
and not having their losses restored. Advocates for the children
say the orphans are more likely to be forced to work long hours,
to suffer from beatings and to experience sexual abuse.

AIDS, however, not only affects the children, it also touches the
new caregivers. As AIDS saps the lives of young adults, family
patterns are reversed. Older people, at a time when they had expectations of their children caring for them, suddenly find themselves becoming caregivers again. In Uganda, Faides Zulu's
situation provides an example of the hardships AIDS is causing
the elderly.

> Faides Zulu, a grandmother from a shanty town outside
> Ndola [Zambia], was supported by her daughter until she
> and her husband both died. Suddenly, Mrs. Zulu had lost
> her only source of income and gained five new dependents.
> Despite her age (she is old enough to have no idea when she
> was born) and frailty, she has resumed the heavy task of
> growing vegetables in her small plot and carrying them to
> market. Hand-outs from a local charity cover clothes and the
> $7–a-year school fees for each child. She says that without
> the 25kg of maize meal she is given each month, the family
> would starve.[27]

The extent of the AIDS problem in the worst-affected communities is pushing the extended family system to the breaking point.
Elderly grandparents, also in need of care, are often the only ones
left to be caregivers. And the death of a grandparent may leave no

one in the extended family willing or able to care for the children, giving rise to orphan-headed households. One study found that in Rakai District, Uganda, children between 12 and 16 years old headed 4 percent of households.

These children, like any child, suffer grief and confusion when they lose a parent. But when AIDS is the killer, the pain is all the more profound. Their loss is often compounded by prejudice and social exclusion, and leads to the loss of education, health care and even property they may be entitled to inherit. The resulting poverty and isolation can create a vicious circle, placing children at greater risk of contracting HIV themselves. In North America, where most of the infected mothers are single parents, no father is around to fill the void. If the mother's drug use has caused her family to spurn her, relatives may be unwilling to care for her children.

Earlier estimates that more than 13 million children worldwide would lose their mothers or both parents to AIDS by the year 2001 were passed by the end of 1999.[28] Today's predictions forecast a threefold increase in that number over the next decade. Zambia, one of the countries hardest hit by AIDS, is becoming known as a nation of AIDS orphans. Having never embraced birth control, Zambia has the highest proportion of orphaned children in the world. An estimated 23 percent of all children under 15 are missing one or both parents, many of them dead from AIDS, and the numbers are expected to keep rising.

For now, most of the children still are being absorbed into extended families. Almost 75 percent of all households are caring for at least one orphan. But with half of all households living in extreme poverty, the strain of caring for extra children is beginning to take its toll. With many more orphans—and fewer working-age adults to support them—surviving relatives are overwhelmed.

Too many think it is a "useless investment" in time, finances and energies when they know children are doomed to die. Others simply believe they do not have the resources or knowledge to care for children with such a devastating illness. As a result many children have no choice but to live out their days alone, caring for themselves as best they can. Children's workers in Kenya estimate that nearly 1,000 AIDS orphans are living and dying miserably on Nairobi's filthy streets.

Many children, like 12-year-old Calvin and 15-year-old Jackson of Zambia, who would like to be soccer stars someday, are losing hope of seeing their dreams fulfilled. Only two weeks after their mother died from AIDS, their aunt took them to the bus station. She said she did not want to take care of them anymore. They were instructed to go to Lusaka, find a police station and ask for an orphanage. But the police could not help them.

As the days went by, the boys slept in rusting, abandoned cars. They had no money or food. This is the plight of countless orphans. As one stated, "Sometimes we are jealous of those who still have parents. It would be nice to have someone who cares about us." Some 90,000 children in Lusaka, like Calvin and Jackson, call the streets their home.[29]

In Zambia, as in most places, when there is not enough to eat, orphans get less food, medical care, clothing and schooling than other children in the household. Advocates for the children say that orphans are also more likely to be forced to work long hours, to suffer beatings and to experience sexual abuse. In the rural areas girls are being married off at 12 or 13. Early marriages mean that the family no longer has to feed the girls and, in keeping with local custom, can claim a bride price.

Even when children are cared for in foster homes, or homes of relatives, discrimination is often evident. Friends may come to visit less often, children may be taunted or harassed by schoolmates, family businesses sometimes lose customers, and children may experience social isolation and not be sent to school. They may be used as servants rather than living as members of the household.

Challenge

There is no doubt that AIDS has forever changed the world for children. Children are often "orphaned" long before parents die, becoming caregivers—and bread earners—for the entire family. Children just eight years old are seen looking after dying parents as well as one, two or three younger siblings. The epidemic has cost them so much. Losing our children to the AIDS epidemic is a price we can no longer afford to pay.

Suzanne LeClerc-Madlala, lecturer at the University of Natal in South Africa, states that "more than anywhere else in the world,

AIDS in Africa was met with apathy." Her reflection on the consequences of Africa's apathy could be true of any continent or nation:

> The consequences of the silence march on: infection soars, stigma hardens, denial hastens death, and the chasm between knowledge and behavior widens. The present disaster could be dwarfed by the woes that loom if Africa's epidemic rages on. The human losses could wreck the region's frail economies, break down civil societies and incite political instability.[30]

As those to whom God has mandated the responsibility to provide compassionate care to the hurting and suffering children of our world, we cannot remain silent. We must vigorously shake off apathy and become actively involved in the children's pain-filled world. United in the body of Christ, we can rise to one of the most urgent challenges confronting church and missions: bringing God's compassionate care and support to children and their families as they face the uniquely painful realities of life in a world with AIDS.

A compassionate response is the only way to make a meaningful difference. Demonstrating Christ's unconditional love and compassionate care restores dignity, gives a sense of self-worth, instills a sense of hope and replaces a spirit of heaviness with the spirit of joy.

Notes

1. Johanna McGeary, "Death Stalks a Continent," *Time* (February 12, 2001), 39.

2. Ibid., 44.

3. The American Association for World Health, *AIDS—End the Silence* (Washington, D.C.: American Association for World Health, 1999), 12.

4. For the most recent statistics, see the UNAIDS and USAID websites.

5. Angus Shaw, "AIDS Decimating Africa," *San Jose Mercury News* (AP) (September 16, 1999), 1.

6. Ibid., 11.

7. For up-to-date statistics, see Children's Cup International Relief, <www.childrenscup.org>.

8. "AIDS Making Africa a Continent of Orphans," Reuters News Media (June 27, 1997).

9. *AIDS—End the Silence*, 12.

10. "HIV-Positive Women in Africa Now Outnumber Infected Men," <www.cnn.com> (November 23, 1999).

11. UNAIDS will publish an update of the latest figures for World AIDS Day (December 1, 2001). For recent published figures, see <www.unaids.org/epidemic_update/report_dec00/index_dec.html>.

12. Ibid.

13. Reported in *Asian Prayer News,* British WEC Worldwide (May/June 2001), 6.

14. *AIDS—End the Silence,* 9.

15. Health Canada, "HIV and AIDS in Canada: Surveillance Report to June 30, 2000" (Ottawa, Ontario), 4.

16. <www.fxb.org>.

17. "Children and AIDS in Thailand: One Country's Response," Stockholm conference, UNAID (August 1996), 1.

18. <www.fxb.org>.

19. The Ministry of Health (HMG), reported in *Today in Nepal* (August 1998), 4.

20. Quoted in Cathie Lyons, "Children and HIV Infection: On Giving Children, Families and the Future a Chance, Focus Paper #11 (New York: United Methodist Church, February 23, 1990), 1. <http:/gbgm-umc.org/health/hivfocus>.

21. Kalinglungliu Gonmei, "Children and HIV/AIDS," *AIDSnet* 2/2 (June/September 1998), 5–6.

22. UNAIDS, report by the Joint United Nations Programme on HIV/AIDS, Brussels (June 27, 1997).

23. "The Role of the Committee on the Rights of the Child and Its Impact on HIV/AIDS: Problems and Prospects," presentation by the World Health Organization Global Programme on AIDS at AIDS and Child Rights: The Impact on the Asia-Pacific Region, Bangkok, Thailand (November 21–26, 1995).

24. Ibid., 2.

25. "Depression in Children with HIV-Infected Mothers May Be Overlooked," Reuters Health Information Systems, New York (October 21, 1998).

26. "Street Children, Substance Use and Health: Training for Street Educators," World Health Organization (1994), 132.

27. "Orphans of the Virus," *The Economist* (August 14, 1999), 35.

28. UNICEF, *The State of the World's Children: 2001.* <www.unicef.org.uk/news/sowc2001.htm>.

29. Suzanne Daley, "Zambia, a Nation of AIDS Orphans," *The Orange County Register* (September 20, 1998), 34.

30. Quoted in McGeary, "Death Stalks a Continent," 53.

2

Clothed with Compassion

Phyllis Kilbourn

> *Thus says the LORD of hosts:*
> *Render true judgments, show kindness and mercy to one another.*
> —Zechariah 7:9

If someone were to ask if we are compassionate persons, most of us wouldn't think twice before emphatically replying, "Yes!" To suggest otherwise would deeply offend us. Of course we feel sorry for those who are hungry, exploited, or abused. After all, we are human, aren't we? But is feeling sorry the same as being compassionate? Will feelings of pity alone drive us out of our comfort zones to an active involvement in the lives of those who are dispossessed, emotionally wounded and marginalized? those whom the world is afraid to touch?

Further, is being human really the same as being compassionate? Isn't our being human the very cause of a whole Pandora's box of evils that continually flood our world? Isn't being human the root cause for the widespread abuse and exploitation of children?

So, what is compassion?

COMPASSION: A CAREGIVER'S GARMENT

Compassion is the all-encompassing garment caregivers must wear to minister effectively to hurting children. We are all familiar with Paul's description of the garments for a warrior going into spiritual warfare (Eph. 6:10–18). Perhaps we are not as familiar with garments God has tailored for those who working with hurting, broken children. These garments are described in Colossians 3:12: "Clothe yourselves with compassion, kindness, humility, meekness, and patience."

Only when the foundational garment of compassion is fully in place will we be able to put on the rest of our caregivers' garments: kindness, humility, meekness, patience. But what is this compassion that is our main garment?

COMPASSION: LOVE IN ACTION

On an outside church notice board I recently read, "Compassion is love in action." Take time to reflect for a few minutes on how you would define compassion or interpret the meaning of the definition just given. You may even want to write down your thoughts. When finished, read Henri Nouwen's definition of campassion and compare it with yours.

> [Compassion] is hard work;
>> it is crying out with those in pain;
>> it is tending the wounds of the poor and caring
>>> for their lives;
>> it is defending the weak and indignantly accusing
>>> those who violate their humanity;
>> it is joining with the oppressed in their struggle
>>> for justice;
>> it is pleading for help, with all possible means,
>>> from any person who has ears to hear and eyes
>>> to see.
>> In short, it is a willingness to lay down our lives
>>> for our friends.[1]

Perhaps after reflecting on Nouwen's definition, many of us would question our initial response. Think about active involvement: crying with, tending wounds, defending the weak, indignantly accusing, joining with, pleading for, laying down our lives. The author further clarifies the task of compassion:

> Compassion asks us to go where it hurts, to enter into places of pain, to share in brokenness, fear, confusion, and anguish.

> Compassion challenges us to cry out with those in misery, to
> mourn with those who are lonely, to weep with those in tears.
> Compassion requires us to be weak with the weak, vulner-
> able with the vulnerable and powerless with the powerless.[2]

In dismay our hearts are probably asserting that such compassion is superhuman. It is! Defined in this way, compassion is not
something we desire to embrace or to which we are attracted. Rather,
it is something that we want to avoid at all costs. And, certainly
compassion is not our natural response to human suffering.

How can we become compassionate caregivers for suffering
children? Compassion can only be transferred to us from the One
who is described as "compassionate and merciful" (James 5:11).
God's own compassion, revealed in Jesus, is our only source of
true compassion. We can only know God as a compassionate God
because the Word "lived among us" (John 1:14). He alone has tasted
fully all our (including the children's!) sorrows and pain. In Christ,
we can share the all-embracing and deeply moving compassion
of God.

BIBLICAL PRECEDENTS FOR COMPASSION

Scripture, from beginning to end, reflects a Father who is the heart
of compassion. In fact, when God was preparing the Israelite nation to know and follow his ways, compassionate living was at
the heart of his rules and instructions. Scripture abounds with
mandates for the care of the widows, orphans and those in poverty. For example, God instructed the Israelites to leave the edges
of their fields unharvested, and to harvest only once and to leave
the crops unharvested one year out of seven—all to provide for
the needs of the poor. They were to be allowed to glean in the
fields without harassment (Exod. 23:11; Lev. 19:10; 23:22; Ruth 2).

The early church went a step further. Its members shared their
resources with the needy and distributed food to widows. This
action sometimes required sacrifice of their own possessions (Acts
4:34–35; 6:1c).

Compassion shaped the ministry of Jesus. Through his compassionate acts of caring, he prepared hearts to respond to the
truth of his message. Each time Scripture records that Jesus "was

27

moved with compassion," that compassion was immediately followed by action to meet human needs. Jesus responded compassionately to the sea of hurting humanity that came seeking his touch: the sick, the lame, the blind, the hungry, the lepers, the widows. He experienced their pain in his own heart. His compassion was love in action.

In every circumstance of need Jesus demonstrated that compassion is broader than a specific function like evangelism or social action. When Christ ministered to people, it was a meeting of the heart and mind that always resulted in answering their needs. His ministry was not simply social action (as in feeding the five thousand) or proclaiming the gospel but a synthesis of both. These functions were interdependent and could not be separated without diluting the effectiveness of Christ's ministry—and ours.

Recipients of Jesus' compassion included children. His heart went out to the woman of Nain, who had lost her only son (Luke 7:11–17). Verse 13 states that "he had compassion for her" and said, "Do not weep." Knowing the value of children in the home and the love between mother and child, Jesus could identify with the mother's pain. He responded to her with a life-giving touch that restored her son to her. He tenderly referred to Jarius's daughter, also needing a life-giving touch, as "child" (Luke 8:54).

COMPASSION AND CAREGIVING

> Blessed be the God and Father of our Lord Jesus Christ, the Father of mercies and the God of all consolation, who consoles us in all our affliction, so that we may be able to console those who are in any affliction with the consolation with which we ourselves are consoled by God. (2 Corinthians 1:3–4)

Children suffering from deep emotional wounds, fear, abandonment, or death need someone to introduce them to the Father of compassion who can heal and restore them, filling the empty voids in their young lives. This introduction initially occurs through compassionate caregivers daily demonstrating the

Father's love. Compassion is a matter of the heart—a necessary ingredient for our ministering life-giving touches to children touched by the tragedy of HIV/AIDS. Only when we feel Christ's pain and sorrow for these children, who suffer broken relationships with family, ostracism by individuals and communities, and a deep sense of hopelessness, along with all the ramifications of their brokenness, will our ministry be infused with compassion. Indeed, we are given the awesome command to be compassionate as our Father is compassionate (Luke 6: 36). That is a tall order, but one for which the Lord is able to equip us.

Geni Crupi, a registered nurse, is an example of God's equipping us for ministry. Geni's first job assignment was on an AIDS unit. It was the last place she wanted to be. But as she began working with the terminally ill AIDS and HIV-positive patients, God began to work in her heart. Geni began to see on the "inside" of these people—what they were experiencing and feeling. God said to her, "You say you love people, so love some of these, society's most rejected." It was then that she realized that HIV/AIDS victims are today's lepers.[3]

And what was Christ's response to the leper? He courageously and compassionately reached out and touched him (Luke 5:13). His commission to us as we minister to those with HIV/AIDS is the same: to reach out with life-giving touches.

True compassion is a work of the Holy Spirit within us. As we expose ourselves to the suffering children and their families experience through the losses and traumas of HIV/AIDS, we make ourselves available for the Holy Spirit to work his compassion into our lives. The Spirit's compassion drives us out of our comfort zones to become involved in a world of deep pain and brokenness, enabling us to demonstrate the love of Jesus to those in need of his compassionate touch.

COMPASSION AND STRATEGIES

The Regional AIDS Interfaith Network's (RAIN) outreach to HIV/AIDS patients through care teams is based on compassionate care. In its newsletter its members summarize their work with the following poem.

> In the pattern of God's purpose, we are stitched
> together in caring and communion: scraps of the
> lingering past, fragments broken from future's
> dearest hopes, textures of disappointments and
> > dreams. . . .
>
> Patched together and transformed into a blanket of
> love. And our compassion comforts a cold and
> hurting world.[4]

Street children suffer much from trying to survive on danger-ous city streets. Their mode of survival puts them in a collision course with HIV/AIDS. Forced into prostitution, pornography and a life of drugs and sex, there is little hope they will escape the impact of AIDS. No one is sure how many street children are in-fected. Testing is usually not available, nor could the children af-ford it if it were.

These desperately needy children are not provided with com-passionate care at any level. They are seen as repulsive and their lifestyle as despicable. How quickly we forget that, for most, they did not choose their lifestyle. Nor is it what God has planned for them. A friend working with the street children in Romania daily demonstrates the compassion of Christ to these children. Recently she sent the following note detailing how a compassionate touch made a difference in the lives of some children living in the most sordid canals of Bucharest.

> Kids from the Brucoveanu metro in the underground canals
> of Bucharest, Romania, are all drug users of a chemical in-
> halant called aurolac. These include Christina and about 30
> other outcasts of the Rumanian society. Christina has been
> on the streets for several years sniffing aurolac. As a result,
> her mind is almost gone. She repeats the same sentences over
> and over. She is tall, beautiful and very kind. . . .
>
> Some Canadian friends recently came over with a doctor
> to give medical help. They spent two days with us in
> Bucharest and came to the metro for Maricica's birthday
> party. Molly, a lady in her 70s, was such an inspiration to
> everyone! She had instant compassion and identification with
> the children. Molly even went down into the canals with

them, gathering courage to descend into the manhole leading to their "home." . . .

At the party, we had cake and cokes and presents for Maricica. We all gathered around Maricica to pray for her, and Molly prayed a prayer that touched and surprised everybody, including Maricica: "Lord, we thank you for this dear young woman. We know that she loves you and wants to know more about you. Bless her in all she does."

Molly didn't see Maricica's faults but instead saw her as she should be and, hopefully, by God's grace, some day will be. It was a great encouragement to Maricica to hear this prayer.

Dear Molly . . . she saw these children through new eyes, through Jesus' eyes. Through eyes of love, hope, compassion and idealism.

God, give us eyes to see clearly every child . . . with eyes of mercy as you see us all. Help us to see wounded children as human—truly human and not as things to be used like trees. Only your touch can give us this kind of vision.

A LITTLE JAM

> I have loved you with an everlasting love;
> therefore with lovingkindness I have drawn you.
> (Jeremiah 31:3, NKJV)

The teacher asked the pupils to tell the meaning of lovingkindness. A little boy jumped up and said, "Well, if I was hungry and someone gave me a piece of bread that would be kindness. But if they put a little jam on it, that would be lovingkindness."[5] What a beautiful description of compassionate care! Not just the basic bread of daily care, enabling a child to exist healthily, adding the jam: joy, hugs, touch, relationships, acceptance, understanding; making the child feel loved, cared for, wanted, of value. This is the jam that changes simply existing to living abundantly. The jam is what richly rewards the caregivers, too, making the task of compassionate caregiving a joy.

Notes

1. Donald P. McNeill, Douglas A. Morrison, and Henri J. M. Nouwen, *Compassion: A Reflection on the Christian Life* (New York: Image Books, Doubleday, 1982), 141.

2. Ibid., 4.

3. Robert E. Logan and Larry Short, *Mobilizing for Compassion: Moving People into Ministry* (Grand Rapids, Mich.: Fleming H. Revell, 1994), 27.

4. Debbie Warren, "RAIN Celebrates Five Years of Compassionate Care," *Raindrops* [Charlotte, N.C.] (Fall 1997), 1.

5. Dr. Sam Martin, *The Arms of Jesus* (Pickering, Ontario), mid term report no. 9 (June 1998), 1.

PART II

The Ministry of Compassionate Response

3

"Your Daughter Has AIDS"

Janice Sakuma

As I looked into the face of my daughter Stefanie, only two days old, her smile revealed two distinct dimples—"cheeks kissed by angels," as someone has said. These dimples, along with the book in her hand, were to be her trademarks. It seemed God had answered my prayers at the birth of each of our three daughters, Penny, Stefanie and then Carin. The girls appeared healthy and normal.

Carin was 6 months and Stefanie was 19 months old. when they were diagnosed with severe factor 7 hemophilia. Because they were missing that factor in their blood coagulation system, clotting during a bleed could not take place unless the missing factor was replaced through blood infusion of plasma or their specific factor concentrate. Stefanie began receiving blood products for joint bleeds when she was 4 years old. Somewhere between the ages of 4 and 8 she was infected with the HIV virus through the blood products she had been given. Although Carin had been given infusions before Stefanie, she needed fewer and miraculously had not been infected.

When Stefanie was nine years old, the verdict was clear: "Your daughter is HIV positive." What incredible pain those words produced. Our world turned upside down for the second time. It was overwhelming to hear that Stefanie would probably die. We had to contend with our initial confusion, followed by tremendous grief, a sense of helplessness and a constant need for hope. Many issues needed to be considered, and many decisions needed to be made.

35

I watched our young daughter suffer and die. Miraculously, I also watched that same child live fully, overcome many obstacles and die with dignity. As a result of this, I can go on living, extending the hand of grace that was extended to me. I share these thoughts in order that you might also become a soothing ointment of hope for those living with HIV/AIDS.

CONFUSION

In 1986, when news of AIDS was unfolding to the US public, the entire hemophilia community was advised to be tested for HIV, Human Immunodeficiency Virus (at that time HTLV III). Both Stefanie and Carin were tested. Carin tested negative, but I was told confidentially that Stefanie had tested positive. Very little was known at that time about this virus, except that it could be fatal. When the doctor said that she did not know if the virus was active, I asked that a test be made to verify whether it was active or not. I did not understand that the disease had three stages of development—asymptomatic (no symptoms), ARC (AIDS-related complex), and full blown—the third stage being considered AIDS. Therefore, when I was informed that Stefanie did not have AIDS (meaning she was not in the full-blown stage), I believed she was not in any danger. I was actually relieved. I felt at peace about the situation.

Besides hemophilia, another significant challenge at the moment was that Stefanie was also living with lupus. In 1987, as the lupus became out of control, Stefanie was sent to a specialist at the UCLA medical clinic. Several tests were run. Then came the phone call and the doctor's words, "Mrs. Sakuma, I have good news and bad news. The good news is that Stefanie does not seem to have any signs of lupus. The bad news is that she is HIV positive in the ARC stage." "Wait a minute," I responded. "I am ecstatic that the lupus has disappeared, but no one has ever been cured of lupus. What happened?" The doctor explained that HIV attacks the immune system while lupus creates an overactive immune system. Perhaps the virus diluted or counterbalanced the effects of the lupus.

"But Stefanie has AIDS?" I asked. "No," he said and explained the progression of the disease. Stefanie was asymptomatic in 1986, but now she was showing symptoms of the disease. Her cell count was below 200, and she was experiencing headaches and night sweats. Stefanie was in the ARC stage of the disease. I cried. The cloud of confusion was clearing and the clarity of the situation was devastating. The active HIV virus was moving Stefanie toward full-blown AIDS and death.

Today I am sure there is still initial confusion when a mother is told her child has AIDS. A whole new world of medical terminology and issues will confront her. Unless she can persevere through the ocean of information, or find assistance, she may drown in despair.

GRIEF AND HARDSHIP

As a child, Stefanie had her own issues to face. How could she find a mode of expression and continue to grow and flourish in the midst of hardship? Through the suffering, her talent for writing, love for reading and fascination with words illuminated the dark times.

> Pain has come upon us . . .
> People may die or be lame
> Pain has come upon us
> Nothing will be the same.

Stefanie wrote those lines at the age of 10. Confronted with the uncertainties of life on earth and the blows of adversity, Stefanie was able to articulate in poetry what she was experiencing. The flow of tears and ink onto the pages of a journal were healthy release valves for her thoughts and feelings. Today her poems have become precious treasures—a legacy and perpetual presence of my daughter.

One of the hardest things I had to do was to tell Stefanie she had tested positive for AIDS. Honesty had always been a foundation of our relationship in coping with hemophilia and the treatments that she needed. So when Stefanie asked to know the results of the test from UCLA, I prayerfully explained the doctor's good news and bad news. We cried together and prayed together. Stefanie had already been exposed to the discriminating attitude of people toward those with AIDS. It was expressed with violence on the news, and she heard the name calling on the playgrounds at school. Children either reflect or fall victims to what adults project and model in any situation or crisis. Stefanie asked: "Can I infect someone else?" "Can I still go to my friends' birthday parties?" What she really was asking was: "Can I still live a normal life? Will I still have friends, still be accepted and loved?" These are still the implications of AIDS, and more so in the early days of 1987. Today, people living in places where there is little knowledge of AIDS and little faith continue to experience fear and discrimination. The depth of despair can easily consume a person.

> We all fall into holes of sorrow.
> We ask a friend to help us out . . .

Grief for Stefanie was the impact of AIDS on her physically, socially and educationally. The loss of physical strength was a major hurdle. Headaches and fatigue were constant companions, forcing her to be put on a shorter schedule at school. This meant less time with her classmates and no after-school activities. Walking to and from the playground required more energy than Stefanie had. She often sat on a wall alone so that she would not be late to class when the bell rang. She was usually the last one through the door at the end of the day because walking had become like moving a ton of bricks. As soon as she reached home, she would take at least a two-hour nap. Warm days took a greater toll; she often looked like a wilted flower. AIDS is a voracious leech that sucks the vitality from its victim.

This vibrant, brilliant child with a zest for living became socially isolated. Her ultimate grief was to having to be home schooled, cut off from her friends. More and more, the hospital with its needles and tests were her "brave new world." This created much sadness for me as a mother. And more and more, her family and church became the warm quilt that God wrapped around her.

The sense of loss begins long before death. Expectation is one area that is affected drastically; we expect to see our children sleep, eat, play, learn, grow, dream, laugh and be carefree. That is a difficult desire to release. How to change the perspective and learn to enjoy life today rather than be consumed by the prospect of death tomorrow was a major lesson God taught me in order to help Stefanie—and me—really live.

Changing the concept of normal is one of the first steps in coping with AIDS or lifelong illness. "Normal" had long ago taken on a new definition for us and for Stefanie. A *normal day* for Stefanie could be five hours in the hospital sitting with her arm on a splint getting treatment intravenously. A *hard day* could be having to be poked several times with the needle to find a vein, having an allergic reaction, or running unending, uncomfortable tests and having to remain overnight in the hospital. An *incredibly good day* was not having to go to the hospital, having the energy to go marketing, bake cookies or visit grandma.

The ups and downs of AIDS are very much like a roller-coaster ride. At her weakest point Stefanie was given AZT, which caused a miracle of new strength. She no longer had to use a wheelchair to get around. She could pick up a pencil and write again. But three months later the drug became toxic and caused Stefanie to become severely anemic. She had to be hospitalized to receive blood transfusions.

Disappointments were constant. The distance in her friendships increased as Stefanie's fatigue meant not returning to school and her Sunday school class, not attending social events or taking piano lessons and studying Japanese. Vacations were cut short and almost eliminated in the end as Stefanie spent more and more time in bed. Her frail body became prone to bedsores, and foods became more difficult to digest. Simple pleasures like a sno-cone or a little note from a friend were pure joy.

As her mother, Stefanie's grief was my tears, her discomfort was my pain, her smile my joy. What a helpless feeling it was to watch her suffer and not have the power to change the situation. How painful it was to see her physical stature diminish, her body waste away as fatigue and loss of body weight reflected the victory of the virus in breaking down her body's defenses and functions. To see death consume Stefanie's young life before its time brought with it the loss of motherly hopes and dreams. I could not imagine life without her. I could not fathom not seeing her grow up, graduate from high school and college, marry and have

39

children of her own. I would not see her become the doctor-missionary she dreamed she could be.

HELPLESSNESS

Feelings of helplessness can lead to hopelessness if the parent and child cannot identify and discern the times when they can control what is happening and when it is out of their control.

For the caregiver and the child, clear information is helpful. The amount of detail depends on the depth of knowledge the person desires in order to cope with AIDS. From the time Stefanie was diagnosed with hemophilia, she was given information about her condition. As she asked questions, we answered them, but we did not give her more information than she needed. Being truthful helped her to understand what was happening to her and to be prepared for what was going to happen. This eased some of the fear of the unknown. Discussing it with her and allowing her to make choices when possible gave her a sense of value and trust.

The one piece of information we withheld was the prediction of Stefanie's death in 6 to 18 months. This would be too great a burden for her to bear. It would have been too great for me did I not believe that the real truth rested in God alone.

Hospitals and doctors can be intimidating. We needed to learn a whole new vocabulary. Procedures and processes are critical for service and survival. Patience is essential to maintaining sanity, and asking questions is the key to empowerment in the health-care system.

Whether child or an adult, people with AIDS are at some time or other dependent on the caregiver for their daily needs—eating, hygiene and mobility. This is when a support system is helpful both for the patient and the caregiver. It was at this time that I had to validate the value of Stefanie's life to her. At one point Stefanie said that she felt sorry for Penny and Carin because they had a sister with AIDS. She needed to know that she was not a burden but a blessing. Total dependence on others understandably can create feelings of being a hardship on others.

Sharing grief helps to remove the barriers of isolation. The listener becomes a companion in what can be a truly rich experience. For Stefanie, journaling in poetry form became her avenue of expression, and I was given the privilege of seeing God do a more powerful work in Stefanie's spirit and heart than the destruction of AIDS.

ISSUES AND DECISIONS

Journaling is a special means of processing and expressing thoughts, but the page cannot take the place of sharing with another person who can listen and be a shoulder to cry on, who can pick up a piece of the burden. However, considering the needs of others was also essential for us. Not only did my husband, Steve, and I need our family and friends, but we also needed to take responsibility for those around us. Who to tell and how to inform them were difficult decisions. Some people deserved to know and have a choice of whether or not to continue to associate with Stefanie, because AIDS carried with it the potential of death.

The doctor advised us not to tell anyone. She believed confidentially was critical to Stefanie's protection. Harassment, discrimination, isolation and rejection were volatile reactions to those with AIDS in the 1980s. However, 2 Corinthians gave different counsel: "By the open statement of the truth we commend ourselves to the conscience of everyone in the sight of God" (2 Cor. 4:2).

This gave us confidence to be open before people who needed to know our situation. Informing our families, friends, school and church resulted in a wider support system for us. Fear of people stigmatizing Stefanie by going public could have limited us from the tremendous amount of grace God bestowed on us. Two verses, Acts 18:9a and 1 John 4:18a, encouraged us during this time and produced a wealth of relationship for Stefanie and for us as a family. People, in times of crisis, need a guiding voice of truth and wisdom, of experience and empathy, to speak to their life.

The first people we chose to tell were our family members— our children, the rest of my family and Steve's family. With our children we set aside a week to take a retreat to San Diego. Allowing each person in the family to understand the situation and acknowledging each person's feelings were stabilizing experiences as we clung to God and relied on him. Although AIDS often scatters families, praying together, and receiving the prayers of others, bound us together.

The enormity of AIDS is traumatizing enough. Add to this the medical terms, medications, specialists and procedures and daily life becomes overwhelming. With the added financial cost and the impact on siblings, it is no wonder that over 70 percent of marriages end in divorce when an illness such as this strikes.

As the end stages drew near, the issue of quality of life versus the longevity became critical. Experimental drugs can produce more daily discomfort than the symptoms of AIDS. Treatments and tests can be continuous and hold so much of the unknown. In the end it was our desire, as well as Stefanie's, to bring her home to spend her last days with the family. "Code blue," using every means of life resuscitation, is a decision that will definitely confront the parents of children with AIDS. What heartbreaking choices these are even when there is faith, hope and acceptance. Yet how incredibly more so they must be without the faith that promises a light at the end of the tunnel.

HOPE

The morning after Stefanie was told she had been infected with the AIDS virus, she brought me a poem entitled "Sorrow." I knew her sorrow was for those who might die without the hope of heaven. But I said to her, "Stefanie, this is a very sad poem. Is this everything you're feeling?" Five minutes later she returned with another poem, "Hope." It reads,

> It is only when you seek
> that you find,
> Some light and hope
> in a wall behind.

> Don't always let walls stand in your way
> in your journey looking for
> a hope or a light
> Keep on going with all your might.

> Keep on going to a land of hope
> A land that lies where no one can see
> And the land that is best
> For you and for me.

Hope is the heart of courage and life itself. With each stage of AIDS comes more loss of bodily function, increasing pain and added medication and tests. Questions plague the sufferer, whether young or old:

Will this misery ever end?
Why has this happened to me?
Is there a reason or purpose to all of this?
If there is a God, why has he allowed this?
Is there something better to look forward to?

The Bible says that Jesus "for the sake of the joy that was set before him endured the cross, disregarding its shame" (Heb. 12:2). The one with AIDS and the caregiver need that hope as an anchor to hold on to as the conditions of the disease ravage the body, creating ever greater isolation and emotional distress. To know that God loves us, has a purpose for our lives and is in control, has provided his Son as a means to rescue us from the clutches of death, and that heaven awaits us can be the miraculous wind that keeps lifting our spirit, keeps the dying and suffering afloat—even flying higher than ever before. This was especially true for Stefanie.

The church and believers have a vital challenge because, in situations like this, we may be "the only Jesus some will ever know." The church and the parents are the transmitters of faith and hope to the child. Stefanie's attitude and perspective were impressed on her by what was modeled by the people around her. It was even more contagious than the AIDS virus and was the difference between living with AIDS and merely dying from it. Premature death in the spirit is a greater tragedy. However, the ability to live so dependent on God each day creates intensity and fullness of life that is beyond comprehension.

I saw Stefanie's spirit rise above hemophilia, lupus and AIDS when she shared with me at low points in my life her own God-infused thoughts. During her struggle with hemophilia and lupus, Stefanie said one evening, "Whenever I am at the hospital and feel afraid, God has given me Psalm 56: 'When I am afraid, I put my trust in You'" (v. 2). I saw her rise above AIDS when she read three books, *The Hiding Place* by Corrie Ten Boom, *Mimosa* by

Amy Carmichael, *Dorie, the Girl Nobody Loved* by Dorie Van Stone. She read these the summer she learned she was infected with HIV. Each was about young girls who suffered but were rescued by faith in Christ. When I said, "What about you, Stefanie? You have suffered a lot." She said, "Oh, Mom, I have never really suffered. I have God and my family who love me."

God intended us to experience his loving presence on a daily basis and to live in meaningful relationship with others. AIDS became the context in which this gift was embraced by our family.

ACCEPTANCE

When I was struggling to accept the prognosis that Stefanie had only a few months to live, Stefanie told me, as we struggled up a hill on a hike, that she didn't like the things that the medication for lupus did to her. But it did make her ankles stronger so she could run and jump for the first time without worrying about a bleed in her joint. Now she didn't have lupus to contend with, but she had AIDS. "You have to give up some to gain some," she said. In that moment God spoke to my fears as her mother. Could I trust him enough to release her to him? Could I give some up to gain some?

My daughters are constant reminders that God has given children the spiritual capacity to know him and live out their faith. Acceptance of what was happening to her became a powerful witness to many people of God's presence in Stefanie's life.

For a mother to accept what is happening and release her child is a major hurdle to overcome. Only God can accomplish this in us. The moment I clearly understood Stefanie had AIDS, and all that implied, I had to accept that I was no longer a mother preparing her child for life only; I also had to prepare her for death. Watching her body going through so many changes was a constant reminder of my own changing role as her mother.

As food for the body became more difficult to digest, food for Stefanie's spirit became more life sustaining. Christ provided grace that was sufficient for each moment. Faith, love, hope, courage and strength came through reading stories from the Bible and books about people who demonstrated courage and faith, who overcame difficult odds. Other sources of strength were songs of faith, physical touch, notes and other acts of kindness, prayers, the testimony of her life, and humor and laughter.

Acceptance and recovery are enhanced when God is made visible in the darkness and confusion of AIDS. First, God's presence is expressed through Christians and the collective body of the church when support and care is given the child and the family living with HIV. Because the death sentence is inherent in the virus, isolation caused by fear can occur even when the patient is among a crowd of people. The human touch can be an act of healing and encouragement. Stefanie was 11 years old when she wrote: "If I didn't know God, I'd have given up a long time ago. . . . He brought people to visit me and pray for me. He gave me new strength each time."

I remember when Steve and I went before our church to inform the members of Stefanie's situation. The tears that were shed, the commitment to stand by us and the prayers spoken on our behalf became a wave of God's grace poured on us. The next Sunday, as many people came up to hug Stefanie, our spirits could not contain the depth of God's love. The human touch was the hand of God breaking down the walls of discrimination and isolation.

God's presence was also expressed through Stefanie's own life. We saw God keep Stefanie's spirit through every affliction; we saw her rise above death itself through Christ as she wrote poems of honesty and faith. Through many disappointments we saw her continue to dream of being a missionary-doctor one day. As her last Christmas gift to God, to her family and to her friends, Stefanie compiled her poems into a book. Today we see how God has fulfilled Stefanie's desire by using her poems to share her experience with people in the hemophilia community, suffering families throughout Japan through The Children of the Stars ministry under Rev. Komatsu, and in churches, classrooms and now this book.

Suffering is redemptive when placed in the hands of God. The result is dignity and value for the life of the child with AIDS, and strength and comfort for the parents and family. In the economy of God I have learned how far-reaching is God's blessing as we collectively suffer and overcome together in preparation for the day of rejoicing when we all stand before our Creator God who has destined us for eternal life.

4

The Church
as Supportive Community

Paul Hudson

The AIDS pandemic, especially in Africa today, has resulted in an explosion of disadvantaged, vulnerable and undereducated children and youth. Caring and compassionate believers in the Lord Jesus Christ have made some tremendous strides in ministry to children and communities affected by AIDS. Most of these believers are in Africa. And though many evangelical churches—even in Africa in the midst of the crisis—remain silent about the problem, some encouraging efforts of believers in our Lord Jesus Christ are yielding results.

One in five adults in Zambia is infected with HIV/AIDS. With a population of 9 million, that means 1.8 million HIV-infected Zambians will die within the next seven to ten years. Many of these are parents, who will leave behind an average of 6 to 9 children when they die. If prevalence and transmission rates continue unchanged at their current levels, a baby born in Zambia today will have a 58 percent chance of eventually dying from AIDS—the highest lifetime risk in the world! Approximately one-third of Zambia's children have already lost one or both parents, and the rate continues to rise.

Even though almost every family in Zambia has experienced the death of a loved one from AIDS, very few are willing to call the disease by its name because of the shame associated with it. Even many Christians see AIDS as a "sinner's disease," beyond the reach of God's grace. But the tide is slowly turning, and some Zambian Christians are putting their faith into action. Their story was told to me by two SIM missionaries working in Zambia, Dr. Bob and Hope Carter, and by Kingsley Kuwema, director of the Mukinge AIDS-prevention program (MAPP) from Mukinge Hospital in Kasempa district, Zambia.

MUKINGE ORPHAN SUPPORT GROUP

Nkunda, the oldest of eight AIDS orphans living with his aging grandmother, was released from Mukinge Mission Hospital with weakness secondary to severe malnutrition. He had been brought to the hospital in urine-drenched clothes because he did not have a spare pair of trousers to wear while his only pair was being washed. His younger siblings and cousins all have very poor growth curves and suffer frequent illnesses. The youngest and most recently orphaned two-year-old child in the family was not able to walk well because of a severe chigger (insect) infestation in both feet. Some other siblings had been missing school because they could not walk due to pain from chigger infestation. The seven year old has a permanent deformity of the hand due to a neglected abscess.

The yard was extremely dirty, partly because the latrine had collapsed and there was no one to help them dig a new one. The grandmother had more than she could manage just to carry a little water for cooking from the well two kilometers away; she couldn't obtain enough water to clean the compound. Even cooking was sometimes more than the old woman could handle, as she was not in good health. Sometimes there was nothing to cook; neither she nor the children were able to cultivate a field to grow their own food. A large tree had crushed their kitchen shelter during a rainstorm a year earlier. The fallen tree was their source of shade and a place for the children to play. But cooking would be difficult during the five-month rainy season without any roof for rain protection. The family had neither intact blankets nor sweaters for warmth at the onset of the cold months.

This grandmother has lost four of her children and their spouses due to AIDS. She has several children who are mentally/psychologically unstable; their whereabouts are unknown. One daughter

47

with six young children, the youngest still an infant, remains in the area while her husband serves a two-year prison sentence. She occasionally attends the church next door but has not been actively involved in a church community. She has no regular source of help.

A ray of hope came into this bleak picture of deprivation when women of the Mukinge Orphan Support Group discovered this family's plight. This group of ten volunteers had already been paying the school fees for some needy primary school children identified by the school's headmaster. They also gathered enough money to pay someone to dig a new latrine for Nkunda's family. Donated blankets and used clothing, including sweaters, were given to all members of the household. The women spent one day cleaning the compound. They also dug chiggers out of feet and cleansed the wounds.

The support group takes food to Nkunda's family periodically and provides transportation to the hospital or clinic for ill family members. It encourages neighbors and other church members to help this family with food and labor as needed. The children now are included in a local orphans' support group, which meets twice monthly for singing, Bible lessons and encouragement. Two women from the Mukinge Orphan Support Group visit at the bimonthly meetings and once in a while in the children's homes, just to find out how everything is going. Once a month the children from five village centers are brought to Mukinge for a video and some fun time. The Mukinge Orphan Support Group is investigating ways to offer other life-skills training and further spiritual support.

The Mukinge Orphan Support Group began early in 1998 when a few Christian women began organizing knitting groups to make blankets for orphans. They saw the great needs of the many orphans in the community and began by giving their own time to pull yarn from old sweaters. The group met weekly for a prayer fellowship. One day they decided to begin canvassing the Mukinge Community for donations to help send a few orphans back to school. Most of the children's relatives simply did not have enough money for even modest school fees. The women received several generous donations, with which they were able to pay school fees for several orphans.

SIM missionary Hope Carter challenged the group to begin an income-generating project to develop their own indigenous source of revenue. Seeds, fertilizer and land were donated to plant maize as a cash crop. Later the group planted three vegetable gardens with seeds sent by missionary supporters. These vegetables are sold locally to raise money for school fees. The orphans help periodically on Saturdays with watering and weeding the garden. Not only does this provide some of the labor, but it also offers experience in gardening and encourages self-reliance. The children realize that they do not always have to be dependent and also feel a sense of accomplishment. Seeds are given to each of the orphan's families for Christmas so that each family can have vegetables and perhaps a little extra income for expenses such as pens, paper and soap.

The women's group is now supporting 90 orphans in five communities, providing school fees, uniforms, pens, pencils and writing notebooks. There is a waiting list of more orphans that need support. With only 10 women, this group cannot take on many more orphans and still provide the personal approach that they feel is important. Their goal is to present the love of God to these children and their families in a tangible way. Rather than just giving money for school fees, they want to get to know each child personally and bring the hope of Jesus Christ into his or her life.

What motivates these women? They have seen the tremendous needs around them and feel called to share the love God has given them. They are all busy mothers, and some have other jobs. There is no material remuneration for them, only the satisfaction that they have helped others. They believe that the "religion that is pure and undefiled before God, the Father, is this: to care for orphans and widows in their distress" (James 1:27). They hope someday to receive more support, but they are determined to proceed anyway until the rest of the community comes alongside to help.

Ultimately, these individuals, motivated by the love of Christ, will make a difference in the lives of these orphans by service, by sharing the gospel of the Lord Jesus Christ, and by genuine concern for the individual children whom they have come to know. AIDS is more than a medical or social problem. Ultimately it is a disease of broken relationships. These women are busy building relationships because of their own relationship with their Lord.

AIDS AND ORPHANS IN KASEMPA DISTRICT, ZAMBIA: BEGINNINGS OF MUKINGE AIDS PREVENTION PROGRAM (MAPP)

Orphans in Kasempa district have always been fostered in the homes of aunts and uncles or other extended family members. This traditional system is consistent with the cultural view that children are members of the entire extended family, not just of one nuclear family unit. However, the impact of AIDS has destabilized the traditional system to the extent that it can no longer fully cope. In some cases AIDS has so decimated extended families that the surviving orphans have no living adult relatives left to care for them. In other cases fostering families have had to take in dozens of children from multiple relatives and been driven into poverty because of insufficient food and finances. Often it is the orphans who are the first to feel the pinch when the foster family lacks access to sufficient food, school fees or health care.

The traditional form of "social security" is for grown children to provide for their elderly parents once they can no longer farm the land, hunt, fish, or provide for their needs in other ways. But now the elderly are outliving their children. Not only are they left without the support they need and expect, but they often find themselves responsible for the care and support of their grandchildren, grandnieces and grandnephews. They cannot carry this burden without the assistance of the community at large. Because most AIDS victims die in their prime, both young and old are left without their traditional source of support, the working adults.

SIM missionary-nurse Jean Williams worked with a team of Zambian national Christians to make a difference. In 1991 she led a hospital team composed of Christians who recognized that there was widespread ignorance and misconceptions about AIDS in the surrounding communities. They began to educate the community leaders about AIDS and HIV infection, beginning with the senior chief and other traditional leaders and opinion-makers. They went into the communities surrounding the hospital, divided into small groups under shade trees, and held group discussions.

50

They began with stories rather than lectures, seeking to ascertain what people already knew about HIV/AIDS. Not surprisingly, the team discovered many misconceptions about the disease. Prevalent among them was the belief that AIDS was caused by bewitchment (witchcraft).

To dispel these misconceptions the team used hospital statistics, including HIV-positivity rates and even mortality statistics to teach community leaders about HIV/AIDS and its prevention. The effort at this early stage focused on the three main ways the disease is transmitted: (1) sexual intercourse (75 percent of transmission is through heterosexual spread), (2) mother-to-child transmission, and (3) exposure to or transfusion with contaminated blood.

Through the use of open-ended questions within the small-group discussion format, community members were led to consider what their roles might be within the context of HIV prevention and the care of those with AIDS. They were asked to identify traditional practices that might spread the AIDS virus, and they were challenged to think of ways they could help their villages face the escalating threat of AIDS. Through it all the team encouraged them to come up with their own creative solutions, recognizing that these individuals would be more successful if the ideas they were implementing were their own.

The base for the Mukinge AIDS Prevention Team was Mukinge Mission Hospital, associated with the Society for International Ministries (SIM) and owned and managed by the Evangelical Church in Zambia. The hospital's vision is to minister to the whole person in the name of Jesus Christ. As such, attending to physical needs and ministering to spiritual needs are perceived as part of the same overall work.

BEGINNINGS OF CHURCH AND COMMUNITY INVOLVEMENT IN THE AIDS AND ORPHAN PROBLEM: THE PROBLEM OF WORLDVIEW

One of the difficulties faced in those early years of the MAPP was the shame and denial associated with AIDS. Believers and unbelievers alike refused to attribute the deaths of relatives to AIDS. Rather, the tendency was to "spiritualize" them, attributing them

51

either to witchcraft or to God's judgment. This had two effects. It kept the people from dealing honestly with the sinful behavior, in cases where that was the root of the problem. It also kept them from dealing in love with the sinner.

In Kasempa the majority of community members are church members as well. It has been said that in Zambia, "when you target the church, you target the community." In this context the AIDS crisis is indeed a church crisis. The fact that there was no discernible difference in HIV prevalence between church members and non-members was a sad witness to the church's apparent moral failures.

Initially, many churches viewed AIDS as God's judgment on those who live sinful lifestyles. Thus they were not interested in becoming involved in ministry to those infected or affected by AIDS—including orphans. But through the persistent efforts of the team from Mukinge, community discussions and correct exposition of the Scriptures (including the many verses about helping the widows, the orphans, the downtrodden and the needy), these churches have completely changed their attitudes and have become actively involved. In the last five years these churches have become a testimony to the grace of God.

Denominational divisions also made it difficult to bring church leaders together and to build unity in the community. In Kasempa there are at least seventeen different denominations. But the magnitude of the problem eventually forced church leaders to come together. As they worked together they were able to overcome many of the divisions among them. Today they even work jointly on other issues. In Kasempa, for example, an interdenominational gathering of church leaders meets monthly to deal not only with AIDS but also with other community problems.

AIDS destroys the body's defense system, but it is more than a medical problem. It is fueled by sexual promiscuity, but it is more than a behavioral problem. It results in families and even villages of orphans, but it is more than a social problem. It is all of these, but it is more. It is a problem of broken relationships. It is a moral problem, an ethical problem. It is a problem of lies and deception. Ultimately, it is a problem of worldview. Dealing with orphans and AIDS in a community means getting to the root cause of a worldview that needs to be changed, renewed and informed by the Word of God.

Our sexuality is designed to reflect God's glory and communicate God's blessings. We cannot control AIDS simply by changing behavior without a change of heart. Sexually transmitted diseases must be controlled by renewed minds, enabled by the transforming power of the gospel. This means men and women renewed in Christ and working for the good of their own family and community, for believers and for unbelievers alike, in the love of Christ.

Not all AIDS is the result of personal sin, of course. It is frequently the result of someone else's sin, or it falls on the innocent. But unless a community deals with the AIDS problem at all levels, including the root level of sexual sin, it cannot ultimately find healing for itself or its children.

Churches in these communities often have not been successful in helping their members apply the transforming power of the cross to their individual lives. There has been much progress, but there still remains an important role for the local churches to play in promoting and modeling holy living, faithfulness, and biblical behavioral standards in their respective communities. The role of moral leadership in the communities should be manifested not only in word, through preaching and teaching, but also in action, through the consistent modeling of biblical standards of behavior in the lives of the churches' members.

Facing the Orphan Problem

Community and church members involved in MAPP began to realize the extent of the orphan problem. The communities were faced with the question of what they should do about the rapidly rising numbers of orphans in their midst. They ended up supporting the traditional fostering system and opposing the institutionalization of orphans.

The rationale behind this was quite straightforward. Institutionalization isolates children from their society and makes them socially rootless. They have no more places in society, no standing, no cultural belonging. But culturally, children "belong" to the whole extended family. This tie is so strong that the paternal uncles are traditionally called Father and the maternal aunts are

53

traditionally called Mother. The villagers, therefore, resist the use of the term *orphan*. The problem, then, is not how to care for a child with no family, but rather how to strengthen the extended family, especially when the adults in it are becoming fewer and older and responsible for excessively large numbers of dependent children.

Brainstorming sessions were held to identify the most important needs of orphans. Two fundamentally different needs were identified: the need for parental love, and the need for financial support. To meet the first need, participants affirmed that orphan children must be full members of their *foster* families, which must consider them and treat them as their very own children. To meet the second need, the participants recognized that the communities themselves had a responsibility to aid and *support the foster families* in their midst to the fullest extent possible.

Community-Based Action

The communities around the hospital have initiated a number of income-generating projects, such as agricultural projects, the baking and selling of scones, and even bee-keeping. Other practical forms of assistance (especially where the caretaker is elderly or infirm) have included collecting firewood, distributing used clothing, cultivating land for planting, and sewing school uniforms for orphan children.

The role of the MAPP program has been primarily to educate and motivate the communities involved, to facilitate community decision-making and the implementation of community activities, to provide technical support where needed and to provide training of community members. This training is tailored to the roles and positions of those involved, including traditional leaders, church leaders, rural health center staff and traditional healers. Each is helped to understand the role he or she plays within the community with respect to the AIDS challenge.

MAPP sought to provide church leaders a forum for the exchange of information, the dissemination of HIV-related knowledge, the promotion of lifestyles consistent with biblical standards, the provision of spiritual ministry and counsel to those living (and dying) with HIV/AIDS, and the definition of the church's role in HIV/AIDS prevention and care and orphan support. Church leaders are encouraged to be in the forefront of community involvement.

While traditional healers are not expected to have a Christian perspective, they do have the confidence of many community members. Consequently, they have been included as a target group for HIV/AIDS education and training. They have responded by assimilating the knowledge they have gained into their practices. In these communities the traditional healers no longer see AIDS as an evidence of bewitchment or the product of a curse, nor do they claim to be able to cure AIDS. Instead, they are actively (and appropriately) referring patients they suspect to be HIV positive to the mission hospital for blood testing. This is a remarkable achievement.

MAPP trains community volunteers to provide home-based care and visitation to those sick with AIDS and to families fostering orphans. Inevitably, some volunteers drop out or become relatively inactive. *Consistently, it is those who are motivated by their Christian commitment who remain the most active and involved.*

Lessons Learned

1. At the community level, care of those infected with HIV and the prevention of HIV transmission are interrelated. One cannot focus on prevention to the exclusion of care. Likewise, the affected children and orphans are part of the community and cannot be ministered to in isolation.

2. In MAPP's experience, income-generating activities in the involved communities are necessary to sustain care and prevention programs.

3. The well-established referral system from the community to the hospital provides a valuable base for the technical support, Christian commitment and prayer for these community initiatives.

4. People living with HIV must be involved as members of the community. Their involvement helps to facilitate the effectiveness of prevention and care activities. Those who are

sustained by a faith in Christ are more willing to accept HIV-positivity and face the reality of their circumstances. They, in turn, are able to help others who have not been able to accept their condition and even, in some cases, lead them to faith in Christ. Those who are able to face their situation from a position of faith in Jesus Christ become some of the most effective counselors in the entire community.

5. Community involvement at all levels is needed right from the very beginning of project design. Even initial planning meetings should involve community members such as church leaders, traditional leaders and other respected members of the community.

6. It is important to care for the caregivers, to provide emotional, psychological, social and economic support where needed. Whether the care is for those suffering from HIV/AIDS or for orphans, the caregivers can burn out if they receive insufficient support. Successful programs must be designed to provide care for those who give care.

7. In the Zambian context, institutionalizing orphans is inappropriate. Instead, there is need to strengthen the ability of the traditional social support system to assist orphans and vulnerable children without removing them from society.

8. Accountability is a problem if funds, equipment and other material resources are seen as belonging to the government or other external agencies. However, this is not as much of a problem if the community itself is seen as having ownership. Those who are responsible for the resources must know they are accountable to the community to which both they *and* the resources belong.

9. Those who are dying of AIDS are particularly open to the gospel, even those who were previously resistant to it. This is why community volunteers are also trained to give spiritual counsel to those who request it. For those who are dying of AIDS, the gospel is the only source of hope.

10. While we encouraged all community members to be volunteers to help their own community members and children, in the end it has been Christians who have had the greatest motivation and made the most impact.

CONCLUSION

The experience of MAPP, from its inception in 1991 until today, confirms the value and effectiveness of the community-based approach to addressing even catastrophic problems of national proportions. It also confirms the value—in fact, the virtual necessity—of involving the church prominently in community-based programs, at least within the Zambian context.

Ministry to children affected by AIDS must be more than a single program. It is possible, with limited resources and reliance on the Lord, to make a substantial difference in a community and affect the lives of children.

PART III

Practical Interventions

5

Longing
for Relationship

Ann Noonan

It is inherent in the human heart to seek relationships with others, and even more important to seek relationship with God. God has designed humans so that in the context of relationships we can take the hand of another and together cross the bridge that securely spans that huge chasm of human fallenness and leads to relationship with God. The bridge is God's own beloved Son, who says, "I am the way, and the truth, and the life. No one comes to the Father except through me. If you know me, you will know my Father also" (John 14:6, 7a). As to our connection with the Father, Jesus told his disciples:

> "If you love me, you will keep my commandments. And I will ask the Father, and he will give you another Advocate, to be with you forever. This is the Spirit of truth, whom the world cannot receive, because it neither sees him nor knows him. You know him, because he abides with you, and he will be in you." (John 14:15–17)

Jesus goes on to say:

> "I have said these things to you while I am still with you. But the Advocate, the Holy Spirit, whom the Father will send in my name, will teach you everything, and remind you of all that I have said to you." (John 14:25–26)

These Scriptures give evidence of the intimate relationship between Jesus Christ and his Father. Also evident is their desire for a relationship with us that could only be given in one way—through the perfect sacrifice of God's only Son for the imperfect ones God created. Knowing us, God realized that we will need an ongoing reminder, teacher, and guide, which God has provided for us through the Holy Spirit. These are evidence of God's love to us, but God has also given us an idea of what he desires from us as an outgrowth of our relationship with him.

Our love for God will result in our obedience to God. To know what that means in the context of relationships with children, we first need to know the mind and heart of God for these little ones.

The Old and New Testaments reflect clearly the value God places on children being properly educated regarding God.

> You shall love the Lord your God with all your heart, and with all your soul, and with all your might. Keep these words that I am commanding you today in your heart. Recite them to your children and talk about them when you are at home and when you are away, when you lie down and when you rise. Bind them as a sign on your hand, fix them as an emblem on your forehead, and write them on the doorposts of your house and on your gates. (Deut. 6:5–9)

God's intent here is that this message needs to be integrated into our lives; we, in turn, need to teach it to our children. I see no exception if that child is not well or not intellectually endowed.

In the New Testament Jesus gives great status to children.

> At that time Jesus said, "I thank you, Father, Lord of heaven and earth, because you have hidden these things from the wise and the intelligent and have revealed them to infants; yes, Father, for such was your gracious will. (Matt 11:25)

At times Jesus would use a child to teach and/or rebuke adults in general and his disciples' poor judgement in particular.

> He called a child, whom he put among them, and said, "Truly I tell you, unless you change and become like children, you

will never enter the kingdom of heaven. Whoever becomes humble like this child is the greatest in the kingdom of heaven. Whoever welcomes one such child in my name welcomes me.

"If any of you put a stumbling block before one of these little ones who believe in me, it would be better for you if a great millstone were fastened around your neck and you were drowned in the depth of the sea." (Matt 18:2–6)

He continues, "Take care that you do not despise one of these little ones; for, I tell you, in heaven their angels continually see the face of my Father in heaven" (Matt. 18:10).

Then little children were being brought to him in order that he might lay his hands on them and pray. The disciples spoke sternly to those who brought them; but Jesus said, "Let the little children come to me, and do not stop them; for it is to such as these that the kingdom of heaven belongs." And he laid his hands on them and went on his way. (Matt. 19:13–15)

Drawing from Scripture we can easily see the premium God places on children. Information from the twentieth century can help us understand how we have gone amiss and/or how we can gain God's perspective. Why does one individual grow up in a neglectful or abusive family and turn out to be a criminal, and another from an equally abusive family become a person who makes significant contributions to society?

I suggest some of the outcome lie in how the individuals experienced relationships. A caring, encouraging relationship can give the child the message that he or she is important, capable of accomplishing important things.

Some of our earliest information regarding the importance of relationships to the development/flourishing of the person was given to us by psychologist Harry Harlow. Harlow's research used monkeys to show that maternal love and close social contacts are necessary at an early age for normal development of behavior. He found that monkeys raised in isolation did not get along well with other monkeys. This was one of the first scientific studies to prove empirically the necessity for relationships for infants to survive and flourish.

One of our deepest needs is to be connected or attached to another. That need begins the moment a child is born. At birth infants begin to get this need met as they are cared for by the adults in their lives. If children cry and someone appears to see if they are hungry or need a diaper changed or to be burped, then they begin to feel safe and secure and that all is well with the world as they know it.

Erik Erikson proposed eight stages of human development that extend through the life span. When a baby's needs are met in a caring way, Erikson's first stage begins to be satisfied—trust vs. mistrust.[1] Erikson's first psychosocial stage is experienced in the first year of life. A sense of trust requires a feeling of physical comfort and a minimal amount of fear and apprehension about the future. Trust in infancy sets the stage for a lifelong expectation that the world will be a good and pleasant place to live.[2] Erikson goes on to say that when a developmental stage is not completed and its tasks accomplished, one can go through life feeling unattached.

It is common to hear people say, "I feel on the outside looking in. I seldom feel accepted by others."[3] Belonging is an awareness of being wanted and accepted, of being cared for and enjoyed. It is the feeling experienced when we sense we are wanted, that we "belong" to some person or a group of people.[4]

Thus our sense of belonging is fundamentally established in infancy. Children develop feelings of belonging when loving parents anticipate their discomforts and affectionately provide for their needs. A tiny infant is sensitive to being loved. When infants are loved in their first year, they develop an essential trust in the goodness of life and the dependability of people. This prepares them for better adjustment in future childhood years and for a happier life.[5] The child has inborn laws of development "which create a succession of potentialities for significant interactions with those who tend him."[6] It is from those around them that infants acquire their view of themselves.

H. Norman Wright illustrated this well in an early book describing how infants develop their self-image. Wright states: "The image a person has of himself *is* determined mostly through his interpersonal relationships. A person's self-image or self-estimate is the result of the *interpretations he makes* of his involvements with others."[7]

The trust that God intends for us to develop during this first year of life will set the stage for our ability to trust in future relationships. The most important future relationship to be developed is the one we acquire at the moment of our salvation experience. So often I have had young and old people tell me they cannot trust God to take care of them, but they can trust God to care for me and others. When we work together, we often discover that this first developmental task has not been met and that this person experienced some trauma and/or rejection during this first year of life. Due to this unmet need, individuals have great difficulty experiencing and believing God loves them. They grow up with a distorted view of themselves and a distorted image of God. This can be rectified through the process of "renewing the mind" (Rom. 12:2) and "putting an end to childish ways" (1 Cor. 13:11), but not without a great deal of work and insight given by the Holy Spirit.

When children have experienced trauma, either in the family or from outside forces, several things happen. They automatically begin to put up walls to protect themselves and often turn inward to create as much safety for themselves as possible. They have learned through their experiences that the world is not a safe place. They shut down their emotional growth while the rest of them continues to develop. This leaves an emotional dwarf/infant inside a growing body.

This lack of emotional development can greatly affect the ability to experience God as a viable person in our lives. What we believe about God in the inner part of us is the most important factor in our lives. If we have experienced severe hurt and/or rejection, as many with HIV/AIDS have, then we probably have difficulty believing the truth about who God is. That God is loving, good, caring—and has a plan for us that is good—is often foreign and difficult to comprehend.

Children who have experienced rejection can only experience healing within the context of a healing relationship. When working with children who are experiencing rejection and abandonment, we need to expect that they are not going to be viewing the world as we do. We need to make every attempt to enter their world and understand how they experience life. When we can do this, we empower the children and give them the message that they are important to the big, powerful people in their lives. It is important that we relate to children from their frame of reference, addressing their needs, and not imposing our own agenda or structure—or our own needs—on them. All children desire relationships, but until we can enter their world and relate to them where they are, we will be doing superficial work rather than authentic soul work.

When children's needs for belonging are not met, they will feel rejection and can even experience difficulty thriving. When children feel accepted and loved, they have a sense of belonging and that all will be well. Their emotional bank account is being filled with positives about themselves and the world they have entered. Conversely, children who are neglected do not develop a sense of belonging. According to the US Department of Health, Education and Welfare (1979), they might reflect any of the following:

- Abandonment—left to fend for themselves either forever or for a long period of time.
- Inadequate supervision or being left alone.
- Involved in activities that are harmful.
- Inadequate medical and dental care.
- Inadequate education.
- Inadequate nutrition.
- Inadequate shelter.

Two pronounced physical conditions that can result from extreme neglect are *nonorganic failure to thrive syndrome* and *psychosocial dwarfism* (PSD). Nonorganic failure to thrive syndrome occurs in infancy. It is characterized by infants who are below the fifth percentile in weight and sometimes in height. PSD can affect children aged eighteen months to sixteen years. These children also show abnormally low growth as well as retarded skeletal maturation and a variety of behavioral problems. Additionally, they tend to have speech difficulties and problems in their social interactions.[8]

Erikson believes that the main theme of life is our quest for identity. Throughout life, we ask ourselves, "Who am I?," and form a different answer at each stage of development. Erikson noted that the process begins when the baby first recognizes its mother and first feels recognized by her. The mother's voice conveys to the child that he or she is somebody with a name and is good.[9]

Stage 2 of Erikson's developmental stages is autonomy *vs.* shame and doubt (roughly two to three years of age). This is a time when children begin to develop some sense of their separateness from their caregivers. If the adults in their life are supportive, they can develop a sense of self-control without a loss of self-esteem. Shame and doubt about self-control and independence come if basic trust has been insufficiently developed or lost. or when children's wills are "broken" by overcontrolling parents.[10]

During Stage 2 limits are initiated and children learn that there are rules that govern their world. When these are given in a positive manner, children avoid a sense of guilt and shame and develop an appropriate sense of autonomy.

Initiative *vs.* guilt (roughly four to five years of age) is Erikson's third developmental stage. The theme of this stage is children's identification with their parents, who are perceived as big, powerful, and intrusive. The basic psychosocial modality is "making," namely, intrusion, taking the initiative, forming and carrying out goals, and competing.[11]

Stage 4 of Erikson's model is industry *vs.* inferiority (roughly 6 years of age to puberty). The great event during this stage is entry into school and developing a sense of accomplishment. Successful experiences give the child a sense of mastery, while failure brings a sense of inadequacy and inferiority. This tends to be a calm period between the first three stages and the next stage.

Stage 5 is identity and repudiation *vs.* identity diffusion (adolescence). This is often thought of as a turbulent period of life for so many things come together for the youngster. "Trust, autonomy, initiative and industry all contribute to the child's identity. The basic task for adolescents is to integrate the various identifications they bring from childhood into a more complete identity. . . . If adolescents cannot integrate their identifications, roles, or selves, they face 'identity diffusion.' The personality is fragmented, lacking a core. Youths seek their true selves through peer groups, clubs, religion, political movements, and so on."[12] These activities give the adolescent an opportunity to try out new roles and experiment in an effort to discover which is his or her fit.

Stage 6 is intimacy and solidarity *vs.* isolation (young adulthood). Only if a reasonably well-integrated identity emerges from Stage 5 can psychological intimacy with other people (or even oneself) be possible. If youth fear they may lose themselves in someone else, they are unable to fuse their identity with someone else. If youths' attempts at intimacy fail, they retreat into isolation. In this case social relationships are stereotyped, cold and empty.

Stage 7 is generativity *vs.* stagnation and self-absorption (middle adulthood). Faith in the future and the ability to care about others seem to be prerequisites for development in this stage. Without these, stagnation and self-absorption, sometimes called self-indulgence, occur. These lead to stagnation and boredom.

Stage 8 is integration *vs.* despair (late adulthood). Acceptance of life's limitations and willingness to face the end of life are aspects of integration. Without these we can end up in despair.

How do we apply Erikson's eight stages of development to children with HIV/AIDS? Youngsters who have not learned to trust due to traumatic experiences and/or rejection will not be able to move on to the next stages. Trust is the undergirding task of all other life tasks. But how can we develop the needed relationships with children to enable them to accomplish the necessary tasks of the early stages?

Virginia Axline's eight basic principles that guide a person entering the child's world of play can be adapted here. She points out that the worker:

1. is genuinely interested in the child and develops a warm, caring relationship.
2. experiences unqualified acceptance of the child as he or she is.

3. creates a feeling of safety and protection in the relationship so the child feels free to explore and express himself or herself completely.
4. is *always* sensitive to the child's feelings and gently reflects those feelings in a manner that develops self-understanding.
5. believes deeply in the child's capacity to act responsibly, within certain boundaries.
6. does not impose his or her agenda on the child but allows the child to lead or choose in the relationship, and resists any urge to direct the child's play or conversation.
7. appreciates the gradual nature of the therapeutic relationship and does not attempt to hurry the process.
8. establishes only those therapeutic limits that help the child accept personal and appropriate relationship responsibility.[13]

In developing a genuine relationship with a child, the adult needs to send the following four messages to the child and live them out in the relationship:

- *I AM HERE.* Nothing will distract me. I will be fully present physically, mentally, and emotionally. I am here for you.
- *I HEAR YOU.* I will listen fully with my ears and eyes to everything about you, what is expressed and what is not expressed. I want to hear you completely.
- *I UNDERSTAND YOU.* I want you to know I understand what you are communicating, feeling, experiencing, and demonstrating through your play, and will work hard to communicate that understanding to you.
- *I CARE ABOUT YOU.* I really do care about the little person you are, and I want you to know that. If I am successful in communicating fully the first three messages, I believe you will know I care.[14]

If children are able to express their feelings and feel accepted, listened to, and understood by a caregiver who is consistent in their life, they may not carry long-lasting effects of trauma. When they are able to feel understood, cared for, listened to and comforted in a healthy manner, the event may not carry the toxicity that is possible when their pain is buried and left inside. I realized an example of this from my own life some time ago. My father and I were talking about a tonsillectomy I had had at age four, and I mentioned that I only had warm feelings about the operation and remembered having had vanilla ice cream in the hospital. He smiled and said, "Ann, that was anything but pleasant for you." Asking him to tell me more revealed a lot about my early relationship with him. He had stayed in the hospital with me and had carried me screaming up and down the hall to comfort me and tell me over and over that it would be all right. I think because of his comfort, not only physically but also emotionally and verbally, I am unable to retrieve anything painful about that memory.

I realize the HIV/AIDS children of the world are in a very different environment from my childhood, but can we not try to reach out to these little ones with the comfort that can only come from God and bear some of their burdens as we seek to imitate their loving Lord and Savior, our bridge between this life and eternity?

Notes

1. Maurice E. Wagner, *The Sensation of Being Somebody* (Grand Rapids, Mich.: Zondervan, 1975), 33.

2. Ibid.

3. Ibid., 34.

4. Ibid., 52.

5. Norman H. Wright, *The Christian Use of Emotional Power* (Old Tappan, N.J.: Revell, 1974), 135.

6. Erik Erikson, *Childhood and Society*, rev. ed. (New York: Ballantine Books, 1969).

7. Wright, *The Christian Use of Emotional Power*, 136.

8. Charles Zastrow and Karen Krist-Ashman, *Understanding Human Behavior and the Social Environment*, 2d ed. (Chicago: Nelson-Hall, 1990), 169.

9. Erikson, *Childhood and Society*, 74.

10. Ibid.

11. Ibid.

12. Ibid.

13. Virginia M. Axline, *Play Therapy,* rev. ed. (New York: Ballantine Books, 1969).

14. Patricia H. Miller, *Theories of Developmental Psychology* (New York: W. H. Freeman and Company, 1983), 163–67.

6

The Healing Role of Touch and Play

Daniel Sweeney

One of the greatest human pains is loneliness. The chronically ill child struggles with this reality constantly. The child is further isolated by the complication and stigma associated with HIV/AIDS. C. E. Moustakas states: "It is the terror of loneliness, not loneliness itself but loneliness anxiety, the fear of being left alone, of being left out, that represents a dominant crisis in the struggle to become a person"[1] We must be willing to enter this lonely place where so many HIV/AIDS victims reside and minister to them.

Consider how Christ would have ministered to the HIV-infected child during his time on earth. Despite the demands placed upon him, he took time to make individual contact with people in need. We know from the Gospels that he did not shy away from people with infectious diseases. He brushed aside his disciples' objections (even rebuking them) when they tried to thwart children from making contact with him and receiving his blessing.

Empathy, arguably the most important skill in the helping professions, was a lifestyle for Christ. And the greatest act of empathy in human history was the Incarnation—God entering our world. Certainly, if it was not below Christ to enter our sinful world, it should not be below us to enter into the fearful and lonely world of the HIV-infected child. Perhaps by entering the child's world of sensation (touch) and creation (play), we learn more about the Creator of all people.

72

Ministry to children with HIV must involve making contact with them in their own world. For children, this world includes physical contact and play.

THE EFFECTS OF PEDIATRIC HIV

The progression of HIV in young children necessitates different and earlier interventions by helpers. Children with AIDS commonly experience several developmental delays, motor disturbances and brain abnormalities.[2] As a result, children with HIV frequently fail to meet typical developmental milestones and may lose developmental abilities after they have been acquired. This often results from an encephalopathy (a brain disease) characteristic of the HIV infection. Neurodevelopmental delays in infants and neuropsychological deficits in older children have been reported in between 75 percent and 90 percent of children with HIV.[3]

Learning and language development are frequently hampered because of the neurological impairments caused by HIV.[4] In terms of language development, infants may experience decreased vocalizations, and older children may lose previously acquired language abilities. HIV children also experience significant decline in visual-motor skills, as well as other cognitive domains.[5]

HIV/AIDS causes significant disruption in the family system. Family members with HIV who have children with the disease may feel overwhelmed, anxious, angry and guilty.[6] These feelings often disrupt the parent-child relationship, which may be further compounded by other psychosocial stressors. The issue of maintaining secrecy about a socially embarrassing medical condition may also place stress on the family. These stresses may result in the child with HIV experiencing a crucial disruption of emotional support when it is most needed.

Additionally, many children with HIV may experience the death of their mother, through whom they contracted the illness. The loneliness of having a chronic illness is then compounded by feelings of abandonment.

TOUCH

The crucial importance of physical touch in the lives of all children cannot be overemphasized. Children with AIDS need it even

73

more. Children are not alone when they are touched; their experience and existence are validated. To be untouched is to be unloved. Certainly, to be untouched is to be alone. Children with HIV are challenged in getting this need met by the family trauma resulting from a chronic illness and then by the unfounded fear many people have of physical contact with a person with HIV.

There is increasing evidence that the skin has an immunologic function.[7] Tactile stimulation has significant positive physiological and emotional effects. Research has demonstrated that separation of infants from their mothers leads to decreased immunological functioning. The classic research by such authors as Rene Spitz and John Bowlby, although not focused on touch, demonstrates this immunological suppression.

The crucial need for tactile stimulation was graphically demonstrated in a simple research study with physically handicapped young children. One group of children was placed on a very smooth surface and another on a highly textured surface. EMG studies showed significant differences between the two groups, with the children on the textured surface showing marked increases in muscle tone.[8]

Nervous system development continues throughout life but is most acute during infancy and early childhood. The type and extent of tactile stimulation received is a major factor in this development. V. S. Clay states:

> The need for peripheral skin stimulation and contact exists throughout life, but it appears to be most intense and crucial in the early phase of reflex attachment. . . . Certainly the young child needs an optimum period for the gratification of his sensual needs, which are both oral and tactile. This is why the preverbal years are considered a critical period for tactile learning. From this time on the needs for tactile contact decline, but tactile stimulation must still be age-graded according to the developmental needs of the human organism.[9]

The medical community is acutely aware of meeting the physiological needs of children with HIV. Tactile needs, and the detriment of failing to meet these needs, are much less obvious and thus frequently overlooked.

The stress and guilt of family members may lead to a decrease in physical touching of the infected child. This may be complicated by ignorance about transmission of HIV, which has prevented many from providing the touch that HIV children so desperately need. There is no scientific evidence establishing touch as a realistic route of transmission.[10] Parents, caregivers and family need to be educated about this. Professionals in the helping professions also need this education. One small study indicated that the majority of professionals in the study had fears about transmission that affected their willingness to interact with the child client.[11]

Tactile stimulation of HIV children may move beyond the important communication of affection and relationship. Some children with HIV develop impairments similar to cerebral palsy, such as spasticity or hypotonia[12] and may need massage and stretching exercises.

Research further demonstrates that there is physiological benefit for both the person being touched and the person doing the touching. D. Krieger's research found that hemoglobin levels increased in both persons, thus increasing oxygenation, which invigorates and can aid in therapeutic regeneration.[13]

The need for children to experience physical touch is paramount. In this age of increased sensitivity to legal and ethical issues of privacy and abuse, however, there is some question as to who should be filling this need for children. My primary recommendation is that parents should be trained in the importance of touch and in appropriate methods for touch. Medical professionals, who are frequently in physical contact with pediatric HIV patients, should be encouraged to include appropriate therapeutic touch to augment necessary medical procedures. Although I do not do so, some mental health professionals include touch as part of their therapeutic approach. This should obviously be done carefully and prayerfully. It is probably best to have any physical contact with children be supervised or videotaped.

PLAY

Play is one of the most important and natural activities of childhood. It is the way in which children process and express their

75

emotional lives. Children need to play to develop emotionally, physically, socially, and spiritually. G. Landreth summarizes the crucial importance of play for children:

> Children's play can be more fully appreciated when recognized as their natural medium of communication. Children express themselves more fully and more directly through self-initiated spontaneous play than they do verbally because they are more comfortable with play. For children to "play out" their experiences and feelings is the most natural dynamic and self-healing process in which children can engage.[14]

Children need to play not only to learn and to develop, but also to make sense of a world that is all too often nonsensical.

Adults are challenged to process the enormity of HIV and its impact on life and family. Children, who developmentally do not have the cognitive and abstract-thinking skills to verbalize like adults, are further challenged to process a very intense and sophisticated issue. They need to have the opportunity to work through thoughts, fears, beliefs and experiences through their natural medium of communication—play. To require children to dialogue verbally about HIV and its effects is not only developmentally inappropriate, but it is yet another unfair imposition on a burdened child.

Since play is a primary occupation of children, it is a significant concern when an illness or disability such as HIV interferes with normal play development.[15] It thus becomes imperative that the adults in the lives of these children create play opportunities for them.

Play therapy may be an important intervention for children with HIV. Levenson and Mellins stress that an important therapeutic goal for HIV children is the expression of emotions and fears.[16] Play therapy, say Cobia, Carney and Waggoner, may provide children with HIV "the opportunity to express their emotions related to fear of death, sense of vulnerability, changes in physical health, and concerns about acceptance from peers and family members."[17] Additionally, McEvoy, Duchon and Schaefer stress the importance of repeated expression of emotions and fears regarding medical procedures and illness for terminally ill children.[18]

Many children with HIV have speech and language delays and disabilities. Speech therapy may be beneficial, but it is equally important to provide these children with play or play therapy in which communication does not depend on verbalization.

Children lack an understanding of illness and death. Preschoolers do not understand the permanence and irreversibility of death and have an unsophisticated sense of causality.[19] School-aged children, while having a greater understanding of the realities of death, are nevertheless vulnerable to fears that the illness or death was somehow caused by something they said, did or thought.[20] The developmental inability and/or fear of speaking about illness and death punctuates the need for a nonverbal experience of play or play therapy.

The benefits of play and play therapy for children with HIV may also be effectively introduced through filial therapy. Filial therapy trains parents to build and enhance the parent-child relationship through play. Developed by Bernard Guerney in the early 1960s, the premise was to train parents of emotionally disturbed children to conduct play sessions at home, thus becoming the primary agent of therapeutic change. Parents obviously have greater understanding of and access to their children than most mental health professionals, making filial therapy an attractive intervention option.

Parents of children diagnosed with HIV, as with other chronic illnesses, are often young and inexperienced at parenting.[21] In a discussion of care for children in critical care settings, C. Rushton notes:

> Parents are overwhelmed with a tremendous sense of not knowing what to do, how to act, or to whom to turn for advice and/or information. Such an experience often threatens the family equilibrium and places serious demands on the parent's resources and coping abilities.[22]

Parents of HIV children not only need access to information and medical support for their children, but also support for themselves.

Filial therapy, traditionally conducted in a group setting, provides an ideal forum for both parent training and the mutual support needed by parents who are experiencing similar emotional turmoil and family upheaval.

Research has demonstrated the efficacy of filial therapy with parents of chronically ill children.[23] These studies reveal a decrease in parental stress, an increase in parental attitudes of acceptance, and a decrease in problematic behaviors as reported by parents.

Readers who are interested in play therapy and filial therapy are encouraged to do further reading and, more important, engage in appropriate training and supervision.[24]

CONCLUSION

It is a natural for those in the helping professions to want to protect and rescue people in pain. It is important to remember, however, that helpers who "wish to be protective need to learn to accept that it is not possible to protect parents and children from all the pain and grief of chronic illness and death."[25] Our task is to help parents and children find resources within themselves to make coping possible. This can be a considerable challenge.

One of the primary challenges in ministering to children with HIV is establishing some level of consistency. Factors contributing to inconsistency and instability for these children include, among others, the emotional turmoil and family chaos inherent in any chronic illness, the change in health and potential decline in functioning and the multiple health professionals involved in treatment. The consistency and predictability that lead to a sense of safety are difficult to find for children with HIV. The task for helpers of these children is to bring them some sense of control in a clearly out-of-control situation.

Consistent physical touch provides not only the benefits noted above but also an anchor to hold onto in a raging sea. Being able to express self through play provides a means to "manage the unmanageable," to control (at least through the metaphors of the play) that which cannot be controlled in reality. These are not therapeutic options; they are necessities.

Moustakas writes: "Sometimes it is necessary for one person to touch another person in his lonely struggle to enable the person to gain the courage and strength to act on his own."[26] We need to touch children, physically and through their world of play, so that their struggle will be less lonely, so it will be filled with the healing power of Christ's love.

Notes

1. C. E. Moustakas, *Portraits of Loneliness and Love* (Englewood Cliffs, N.J.: Prentice-Hall. 1974), 16.

2. S. Kalichman, *Understanding AIDS: A Guide for Mental Health Professionals* (Washington, D.C.: American Psychological Association, 1995); B. Lowenthal, "Pediatric HIV Infection: Effects on Development, Learning, and Interventions," *Early Child Development and Care*, 136 (1997): 17–26.

3. J. Adnopoz, B. Forsyth, and S. Nagler, "Psychiatric Aspects of HIV Infection and AIDS on the Family," *Child and Adolescent Psychiatric Clinics of North America*, 3/3 (1994): 543–55.

4. J. Hanna, and M. Mintz, "Neurological and Neurodevelopmental Functioning in Pediatric HIV Infection," in *Children, Families, and HIV/ AIDS*, ed. N. Franklin, G. Steiner and M. Boland (New York: Guilford Press, 1995).

5. E. Frank, G. Foley and A. Kuchuk, "Cognitive Functioning in School-age Children with Human Immunodeficiency Virus," *Perceptual and Motor Skills*, 85/1 (1997): 267–72.

6. Adnopoz et al., "Psychiatric Aspects of HIV Infection and AIDS on the Family"; Lowenthal, "Pediatric HIV Infection."

7. A. Montagu, *Touching: The Human Significance of the Skin* (New York: Harper & Row, 1986).

8. L. Linkous and R. Stutts, "Passive Tactile Stimulation Effects on the Muscle Tone of Hypotonic Developmentally Delayed Young Children," *Perceptual and Motor Skills* 1/3 (1990): 951–54.

9. V. S. Clay, "The Effect of Culture on Mother-Child Tactile Communication," *Dissertation Abstracts International* 28/05 [AAT 6705537] (1966), 308.

10. J. Landau-Stanton and C. Clements, *Aids, Health, and Mental Health: A Primary Sourcebook* (New York: Brunner/Mazel Publishers, 1993).

11. N. Lopez-Reyna, R. Boldman and J. Kahn, "'Professionals': Perceptions of HIV in an Early Childhood Developmental Center," *Infant-Toddler Intervention*, 2/6 (1996): 105–16.

12. Lowenthal, "Pediatric HIV Infection: Effects on Development, Learning, and Interventions."

13. D. Krieger, "Therapeutic Touch: The Imprimatur of Nursing," *American Journal of Nursing* 75/5 (1975), 784–87.

14. G. Landreth, *Play Therapy: The Art of the Relationship* (Muncie, Ind.: Accelerated Development Press, 1991), 10.

15. R. Parks, F. Oakley and M. Fonseca, "Play Development in Children with HIV Infection: A Pilot Study," *American Journal of Occupational Therapy* 52/8 (1998), 672–75.

16. R. Levenson and C. Mellins, "Pediatric HIV Disease: What Psychologists Meed to Know," *Professional Psychology and Practice* 23 (1992): 410–15.

17. D. Cobia, J. Carney and I. Waggoner, "Children and Adolescents with HIV Disease: Implications for School Counselors," *Professional School Counseling* 1/5 (1998): 43.

18. M. McEvoy, D. Duchon and D. Schaefer, "Therapeutic Play Group for Patients and Siblings in a Pediatric Oncology Ambulatory Care Unit," *Topics in Clinical Nursing* 7/1 (1985): 10–18.

19. M. Speece and S. Brent, "The Development of Children's Understanding of Death," in *Handbook of Childhood Death and Bereavement*, ed. C. Corr and D. Corr (New York: Springer Publishing Co., 1996); N. B. Webb, "Assessment of the Bereaved Child," in *Helping Bereaved Children: A Handbook for Practitioners*, ed. N. B. Webb (New York: Guilford Press, 1993).

20. J. Le Vieux, "Group Play Therapy with Grieving Children," in *Handbook of Group Play Therapy*, ed. D. Sweeney and L. Homeyer (San Francisco: Jossey-Bass Publishers, 1999).

21. D. Cherry, "Stress and Coping in Families with Ill or Disabled Children: Application of a Model to Pediatric Therapy," *Physical and Occupational Therapy in Pediatrics* 9/2 (1989): 11–32.

22. C. Rushton, "Family-centered Care in the Critical Care Setting: Myth or Reality?," *Children's Health Care* 19/2 (1990): 68.

23. H. Glazer-Waldman, J. Zimmerman, G. Landreth and D. Norton, "Filial Therapy: An Intervention for Parents of Children with Chronic Illness," *International Journal of Play Therapy* 1/1 (1992): 31–42; K. Tew, "The Efficacy of Filial Therapy with Families with Chronically Ill Children," *Dissertation Abstracts International* 58/03 [AAT 9727806], (1997).

24. For further information on play therapy and filial therapy, see D. Sweeney, *Counseling Children Through the World of Play* (Wheaton, Ill.: Tyndale House Publishers, 1997); Landreth, *Play Therapy: The Art of the Relationship*; and Rise Van Fleet and Louise Guerney, *Casebook of Filial Therapy* (Play Therapy Press, in press). For training on play therapy and filial therapy, contact the Center for Play Therapy, 940–565–3864 or

<www.coe.unt.edu/cpt/> or the National Institute for Relationship Enhancement, 800–4–FAMILIES or <www.nire.org>

25. R. Bor, R. Miller and E. Goldman, *Theory and Practice of HIV Counseling: A Systemic Approach* (New York: Brunner/Mazel Publishers, 1992), 116.

26. Moustakas, *Portraits of Loneliness and Love.*

7

Binding Up
the Brokenhearted Child

Snowden Albright Howe

Everyone old enough to love is old enough to grieve.[1] Children are not immune to the pain of grief, especially to the immense grief that can follow the death of one who is *especially* loved such as a parent (or parents!), a sibling, or any other close relative or friend. In the presence of worldwide HIV/AIDS epidemics, such grief experiences are all too common. How can compassionate caregivers best help grieving children so that their pain can be an avenue for growth rather than a pathway to adult dysfunction or even psychopathology?

Phyllis Kilbourn suggests a perspective that can apply to any emergency situations—war, abuse, HIV/AIDS, and/or profound loss and grief—that confront children around the world:

> It has been proven . . . that intervention by committed, lov-ing caregivers who recognize that the children's future growth and development depend on successfully interven-ing in their emergency situations can enable children to pass through these intense crises with a strengthened sense of self, a renewed trust in their coping skills and a firmer faith in the love and care of their Heavenly Father.[2]

These truly are significant goals. And they offer the possibility of hope in the midst of crisis, a biblical perspective that "we know that all things work together for good for those who love God, who are called according to his purpose" (Rom. 8:28).

A similar view is found in Granger Westberg's *Good Grief.*[3] In this small book Westberg suggests that people often take the scriptural command to "grieve not" out of context, which is to "not grieve as others do *who have no hope*" (1 Thess. 4:13, italics added). Perhaps the major job facing compassionate caregivers who work with grieving children is to provide the *hope*—and the help—that is needed for the grief experience to be seen eventually as "good grief." Out of their experience of loss, the children may one day grow stronger in themselves, in their relationship to God, and perhaps in their ability to help others.

HELPING HEALING RELATIONSHIPS

> When a loved one dies, children grieve. The most important factor in how children react to the death is the response of the adults who influence their lives. . . . The challenge is to learn how to establish *helping-healing* relationships with children whose lives have been touched by the death of a loved one. When caring adults meet his challenge, children are capable of reconciling grief in healthy ways.[4]

How can these "helping-healing relationships"—the heart, in fact, of compassionate caregiving—be established when children are grieving? In *A Child's View of Grief*, often supplied by funeral homes, Dr. Wolfelt applies four basic components of caring relationships to grief situations: respect, acceptance, warmth and understanding.

Respect is conveyed by treating each child as a unique individual, able to determine what his or her needs are and how best to meet them. Adults would rarely go to other adults in a time of loss and tell them that they should or shouldn't cry, should or shouldn't attend the funeral, should be quieter, should not yell, should leave the room, should talk about the loss right then, should not talk about the loss right then, and so on. Such behavior would not demonstrate respect for or confidence in grieving persons' ability to know themselves and to make wise decisions! Adults, however, often attempt to make similar decisions for children in crisis. In the words of children:

> "I wish grown-ups would let me tell them something. It just seems like all the adults talk to me since my mommy died, but they don't let me talk."

> "If you assume you know all about my grief; it's like you don't respect me. The love I had for the person who died was very special and not like anybody else's. And I'm differ-ent—nobody else is just like me. It's all right if you try to understand how I feel, but please don't tell me you know just how I feel because you don't. All I need is for you to help me find ways to tell you how I feel and for you to really listen to me."[5]

Closely linked to respect is *acceptance*—acceptance of whatever means the child chooses to cope with the loss. Grief can involve many emotions, sometimes conflicting emotions, sometimes emo-tions that are not "nice." Grief involves many stages. These emo-tions and stages will be examined later, but it is important for children to be able to express whatever they are feeling without fear of judgment or disapproval. In a child's words, "We need to share our grief without fear of being criticized or abandoned.[6]

Warmth is another crucial element in helping-healing relation-ships and an essential aid for grieving children. It has been said that two-thirds of all communication is nonverbal,[7] and most chil-dren are far more skilled at interpreting nonverbal messages than are adults. Children *know* when adults genuinely care about them; genuine caring is probably what children—and adults—need most at a time of loss. This is expressed well by Norman Vincent Peale:

> The best antidote for sorrow is affection, caring, love. And the best way to help a person in grief is to express those things in any way that you can.
>
> I shall never forget the second funeral I had to conduct as a young minister. A little girl had died. She was about 8 years old. I can still remember her, lying in her casket as if asleep, with pink ribbons in her hair. The young parents sat nearby,

stunned with grief. I was so young and inexperienced myself that I seriously doubted my ability to conduct the service without breaking down. So before it began, I did the only thing I could think of. I went over and sat between the father and the mother and put my arms around them and told them, through the tightness in my throat, that I loved them. Later the mother told me that this gesture touched and helped her more than anything I could have said or done.[8]

Warmth and genuine caring are especially needed when grief occurs, and warmth can be expressed through behavior, tone of voice, eye contact, posture and facial gestures as well as through words.

Understanding is also needed in effective helping-healing relationships. Understanding can grow out of the relationship characteristics already mentioned: respect, acceptance and warmth. As in a circle, when a grieving child's words, actions and feelings are respected and accepted with warmth and genuine caring, the child is able to express himself or herself more freely, and the caregiver's understanding of the child increases. The helper is therefore able to express more genuine respect, acceptance and warmth, and the relational circle continues. Most adults have experienced this cycle of increased understanding and relationship closeness. In fact, most can remember times when that closeness seemed to be a lifesaver. Children need these helping-healing relationships, especially when someone who has been a major source of love, understanding and support has been removed from their world through death. They need the nonverbal message that even though that loved one will not return, there can be other relationships in their lives that also will give them acceptance, warmth and understanding. This provides hope.

EXPLAINING DEATH TO CHILDREN

Some of the most significant guidelines for discussing death with children may seem obvious, but they are often overlooked. The most important of these is the need for *honesty*. As already stated, children are adept at nonverbal communication; they are able to recognize the feelings and uncertainties adults may not be putting into words. Caregivers at a time of grief will be much more able to help others if they have done their own grief work in the past. An honest "I don't know, but we can think or talk or ask others," is usually better received by children than a made-up or half-true answer. Adults are less than honest sometimes because they think they are protecting children by shielding them from painful realities; often, however, the "answers" that children's imaginations then supply are more difficult for the children to handle than the facts would have been.[9]

While honesty is essential, *simplicity* is also important. Caregivers should listen carefully to children's questions so they can provide only the amount of information they are really seeking at the time. An uncomfortable adult has a tendency to provide far too little—or far too much—information about emotion-laden topics such as death or sex. When children feel safe with an adult and sense that their questions will be answered honestly, they will return as often as necessary to get the information or reassurance they seek. In fact, grieving children often need to repeat questions several times before they can fully process the answers.

Keeping answers *age-appropriate* is also very important. Younger children may especially have difficulty understanding adult expressions. When a school nurse died, a teacher told the class, "I'm sorry to tell you, but we lost Mrs. Thompson." A student replied, "Don't worry. We'll find her."[10]

Children often mistake the meanings of words and phrases. "I was once asked by a young girl, 'How long is death?' I responded, 'Death is permanent.' The youngster said, 'Oh, then it's not so bad.' Noticing my bewilderment she said simply, 'My mother has permanents at the hairdresser. It doesn't last very long.'"[11]

Other misunderstandings are less humorous and more troubling. When children are told that a deceased loved one is "sleeping," they may be afraid to fall asleep themselves. Similarly, if a terminal illness is not explained clearly, children may fear that they—or other loved ones—are in danger of immediate death every time they become sick. The common explanation that a loved one is on a "journey" or has "gone away for a long time" may create unnecessary hurt or anger in the child because it sounds *voluntary*.[12]

Euphemisms involving God may also cause serious problems for children as they grow older. For example, "God wanted your daddy in heaven with him because he was such a good man," could cause resentment toward God or fear of also being "good and wanted by God." It could lead to a conviction that death happens only to some special people and not to everyone.[13]

One of the goals in explaining death to children is to construct a solid foundation of information—honest, simple and age-appropriate—that can be built upon as the children mature. Even the wisest adults do not have all the answers about death and dying; there is no reason to pretend to have them all or to create make-believe or overly simple explanations that will have to be adjusted later. If compassionate caregivers can provide a foundation of trust and truth for grieving children, then children will be able to continue that growth in trust and truth as they mature.

Helping children understand death, however, is only part of a caregiver's task; helping children through their emotional reactions to death is probably far more significant and certainly more challenging. To help children, adults need an understanding of the emotions and stages that may occur throughout the grieving process.

UNDERSTANDING THE GRIEF PROCESS

Dr. Elisabeth Kubler-Ross, widely recognized as a pioneer and leading authority on death and dying, has identified five stages through which people pass as they attempt to come to terms with death.[14] These stages are the same whether people are faced with their own impending death or the death of a loved one. The stages, however, do not necessarily occur uniquely or chronologically; they may occur repeatedly and in any order. These stages are not to be used to designate a person's "progress" through the grieving process. Instead, knowledge of the stages and of the varying emotions that accompany them can provide a basis for the understanding, acceptance, respect and support that were discussed earlier as critical components in helping-healing relationships.

PRACTICAL INTERVENTIONS

Stage #1: Denial

Denial is, as Dr. Kubler-Ross says, the "No, not me!" stage. Denial is often understood by adults; it is a God-given numbness by which we are temporarily protected from the impact of a great shock. Adults, however, are slower to recognize denial in children; they assume that children are too young to grieve or too self-absorbed or will quickly forget the loss. In fact, children may be simply moving in and out of the stage of denial as a way of protecting themselves from too much pain—the same process that occurs with adults.

Children may *act out* this stage in different ways than adults do: they may laugh or be very loud and noisy; they may return quickly to their play (or other distractions) as if nothing has happened; or they may demonstrate an apparent lack of feelings. Just as an adult puts a Band-Aid on a child's physical wound, adults must respect a child's need to temporarily cover up emotional wounds.[15]

Stage #2: Anger

Another stage is *anger*, the "Why me?" stage. This stage is explained to adults as follows:

> Almost everyone experiences anger when faced with the loss of a loved one. That anger is often expressed toward others, sometimes with reason, sometimes without. . . . We often express that anger toward family and friends, resulting in many a ruptured relationship. We might turn the anger in upon ourselves, berating ourselves for some unspoken word, some unresolved conflict. And we all must admit that at times we are angry with God. Yes, even believers can feel anger toward God for their loss, and anyone who denies this simply isn't being honest. Thankfully God is big enough to handle our anger and our tough questions. We should also mention the fact that, surprising as it is to many, there are folks who feel anger *toward the person who has died.*[16]

It is important to note, however, that

> the bereaved are often bitter and resentful for their misfortune; they may become irritable and difficult to manage. . . .

> A first impulse of an enraged individual is to lash out. . . .
> Adults understand this need to vent their hostility, yet often
> they won't tolerate this behavior in their children.[17]

> This dimension of grief (explosive emotions) is often the most
> upsetting for adults. Parents and others are uncertain how
> to respond to an expression of complex emotions such as
> anger, blame, hatred, terror, resentment, rage and jealousy.
> Behind these explosive feelings, however, are a child's more
> primary feelings of pain, helplessness, frustration, fear and
> hurt caused by the death of a loved one.[18]

Closely related to anger, but often not recognized as such, are feelings of *irritability* (being emotionally vulnerable, easily offended, hurt)[19] and *acting-out behavior* (temper tantrums, rebellion, fighting, or even an "I don't care" attitude).[20] Also in this "negative emotion" stage, there may be feelings of shame, blame and guilt.

> Children often experience shame, blame or guilt after the
> death of a loved one because they have directed their natu-
> ral anger from their loss inward. Adults at times may blame
> themselves for a death: "If only I had talked to him more
> about my values" or "If only I had not let her go there that
> night." But the process becomes more complicated with chil-
> dren because they may easily misunderstand the ways that
> death can occur, and they may apply "magical thinking" to
> the problem. A child, for example, who screams at a parent,
> "I'm so mad at you! I hope you die!" may truly believe that
> his words had a major influence on the parent's illness or
> death. Or children may incorrectly determine that their ac-
> tions caused a loved one's death.[21]

Children, like adults, may feel guilty about ways they interacted with the loved one before the death occurred; they may have regrets about things they said or did—or failed to say or do. When it is too late to say, "I'm sorry," these memories may take on a magnified importance; those who are grieving may need reassurance ("No one is perfect, and look at all the ways you *did* make your dad happy."). And they may need gentle reminders of God's grace and willingness to forgive.

Guilt may also occur when anger is directed at God or at the deceased loved one. As stated earlier, people do not like to confess that they are blaming God for the death or that they are angry at their loved one for being careless or for catching the fatal illness and thereby "deserting" them in death. When children hide their anger because they believe they are "bad" to have those feelings, they must then struggle with guilt or shame as well as anger.

When the depth and variety of these anger-related emotions are considered, it is easy to see why a healing-helping relationship with a grieving child is of such importance. Children will only feel safe enough to put these "bad" feelings into words when they trust a caregiver to treat them with respect, acceptance, understanding and warmth. And being able to express these feelings within a trusting relationship is one of the best ways to work through the negativity and move toward healing.

Stage #3: Bargaining

Stage three, *bargaining*, the "Yes, me, *but* . . . " stage will be discussed only briefly, because it seems to be more applicable before, rather than after, a death. When facing a terminal illness in themselves or a loved one, children (and adults) sometimes make promises (often not kept later) to God—or perhaps to the doctor—about what they will do if a special request is granted. An example might be the child who prays, "Dear God, I will never be mean to my sister again if you just let my mommy live till my birthday."

This bargaining stage is particularly significant to caregivers if they need to help children work through their anger or guilt on the other side of these promises. The boy whose mommy did live until his birthday, for example, but who is now venting his grief at her death through meanness to his sister, may have a difficult struggle with guilt. "Survivor guilt" is a related phenomenon in which a person feels bad that he or she is still alive and the "better" sibling or "Daddy who took care of us" is not alive.

Stage #4: Depression

There is *depression*, the "Yes, me" stage. This is the time when one can no longer deny, bargain away, or run in anger from the fact of death. (Remember, these stages do not necessarily occur in this

90

order, and each stage can be revisited any number of times.) In *Good Grief* Westburg writes:

> Eventually there comes a feeling of utter depression and iso-
> lation. . . . When we find ourselves in the depths of despair
> . . . we would remind ourselves that this is to be expected
> following any significant loss, and that such depression is
> normal and a part of good healthy grief. One way to describe
> a depression is to say it is much like a very dark day when
> the clouds have so blacked out the sun that everyone says,
> "The sun isn't shining today." We know that the sun is shin-
> ing, but it appears as if it is not. . . . This is what a depression
> is like. Something seems to come between the person and
> God and between the person and his fellow man, so that he
> feels a tremendous loneliness, an awful sense of isolation.
> And he can't seem to break through it.[22]

In Roberta Temes's *The Empty Place,* a little boy relates:

> In my family there is an empty place
> There is an empty place in the kitchen
> In the backyard,
> Even in the car.
> Sometimes I feel an empty place inside me, too.
> When I feel empty, the emptiness is in the middle of my heart.
> Sometimes I am a regular, ordinary third-grader,
> But some days, I feel sad, or I feel lonely, or I feel sorry, or I
> feel . . . scared[23]

An important consideration in this stage is the role of tears. Dr. Grollman provides helpful insight:

> Tears are a tender tribute of yearning affection for those who
> have died but are not forgotten. Weeping helps to assuage
> heartache—to express that inevitable depth of despair that
> follows the slow realization that the death is not a bad dream.
>
> Do not be afraid of causing tears; they are like a safety
> valve. Often people deliberately turn a conversation away
> from loss. They are apprehensive of the weeping that may
> follow. They do not understand that expressing grief is nor-
> mal and helpful. . . .

> While you should not deny a youngster the opportunity to weep, neither should you urge the child to display unfelt feelings. . . . Each child reacts differently. Some children need to cry freely. Others may be able to get by with a few tears. . . . There are other outlets for emotions besides tears. Allow them to express those feelings that are appropriate to their needs.[24]

In addition to sadness and loneliness, children may also experience feelings of *fear* and *anxiety*. As the reality of death becomes apparent to them, they begin to worry about who else might die. And as the foundation of their world is shaken, they worry about what will change next. They may ask, "Mommy, are you going to die, too? Who will take care of me? What is going to happen to me now?" These fears are repeatedly expressed in a book by Jill Krementz, *How It Feels When a Parent Dies*.[25] This book consists of photographs and interviews with eighteen children from ages seven to sixteen who candidly discussed their reactions to a parent's death. There are two recurring themes in their comments. The first involves fears about how life will change. Will we have enough money now? Will we have to move? Who will pick me up from school? And the second fear is about the possibility of their own or other people's deaths. These young people were also, quite naturally, concerned about the reactions of friends. Will they treat me differently? Will they feel sorry for me? Will they still play with me? They seemed eager for life to become as normal again as possible without shattered innocence and without anxiety about what other terrible thing could occur.

Throughout the grieving process, in any of the stages, there may be physical as well as emotional responses to loss. Children may lose their appetites, become unable to sleep, or complain of upset stomachs or headaches. Children may also show signs of regression such as bed-wetting or thumb-sucking. They may demonstrate hyperactivity or an inability to concentrate. They may begin clinging to family members out of fear of separation, or they may withdraw from loved ones in an attempt to avoid the possibility of further hurt or loss. In the same ways that respect, acceptance, warmth and understanding provide a child with a safe environment in which to express negative emotions, these aspects of a caring relationship also allow a child to express and thereby "get beyond" these negative behaviors that grow out of grief.

Stage #5: Acceptance

The stage of *acceptance* shows a change in focus away from the past and toward a future in which hope again plays a part. Dr. Wolfelt calls this stage "reconciliation" and says:

> While children never get over their grief, they become reconciled to it. At this point, children recognize life will be different without the presence of the person who has died. Yet they have a renewed sense of energy and confidence and want to become involved in the activities of life again.[26]

And Dr. William Worden, writing about "successful grieving," states:

> Successful grieving helps a person to: (1) accept the reality of the loss, (2) experience the pain of grief, (3) adjust to an environment in which the deceased is missing, and (4) withdraw emotional energy and reinvest it in another relationship.[27]

Especially helpful is a chart by Dr. H. Norman Wright:[28]

Loss-Hurt	*Loss-Adjustment*
shock	helping others
numbness	affirmation
denial	hope
emotional outbursts	new patterns
anger	new strengths
fear	new relationships
searchings	"re-entry" troubles
disorganization	depression
panic	loneliness
guilt	isolation

PRACTICAL INTERVENTIONS

Obviously, compassionate caregivers want to help grieving children come up out of the "valley," to look forward to new relationships, new strengths and renewed hope for the future. Helping-healing relationships work to promote increased understanding of both death itself and the grieving process.

TOOLS FOR RECOVERY

It is helpful to offer those who are grieving the opportunity to express their pain in a number of ways. *Art* is, naturally, a medium for symbolic nonverbal language, and many children will also demonstrate their feelings and concerns through the symbolic nonverbal language of *play*. *Journals* and other *creative writing* opportunities may encourage the use of symbolic verbal language as a means of releasing some of the grief; sharing *literature* that deals with death in symbolic or nonsymbolic terms may also aid children in expressing their feelings. *Support groups* in which children can talk with others who have suffered similar losses have been found by many to be very helpful avenues for healing. And some people have been aided through their grief by *commemorating* the loved one. Suggestions and examples follow for each of these specific tools for healing.

Art, with its use of symbolic nonverbal language, can provide a powerful tool for healing. People in pain—at any age—often put into pictures things that are too scary or traumatic to express in words. Caregivers can provide children with large pieces of paper and any art medium available (pencils, paint, crayons, markers); clay or sand can also be used. Children should be encouraged to create whatever they choose, and then they should be encouraged to explain their own art, *if* they choose to do so.

In her tapes Dr. Kubler-Ross tells about a terminally ill child who drew two pictures. The first showed a huge army tank bearing down on a tiny person holding a stop sign (probably indicating the helplessness the child felt in relation to the illness). Dr. Kubler-Ross points out that if a child shares a picture like this with an adult, it may indicate a readiness on the child's part to discuss his or her concerns with that adult. After Dr. Kubler-Ross encouraged the child to put into words the feelings expressed in the first picture, the child then drew a bird with a gold-tipped

94

wing. When Dr. Kubler-Ross asked the child to explain this picture, she said, "Can't you see? It is a peace bird" with the "sunshine of heaven on its wing." Communicating through symbolic nonverbal and then verbal language allowed this child to come to better terms with her impending death.

Play can also provide children with a means of expressing grief. One child, for example, when playing with a doll house and a small family of dolls, "acted out" his father's death by repeatedly removing the daddy doll and "flying" him to the roof of the play house. On several occasions he also took the small boy doll and placed him on the roof with the daddy; this was a child who had been brought to therapy because his mother was concerned that he was contemplating suicide due to his grief about his dad (actual case history). In some cases play can be used as a springboard to conversation; in other cases play can be seen as therapeutic in itself as the child "works through" issues nonverbally.[29]

Journaling and creative writing have long been recognized by therapists as excellent methods of helping clients work through grief and/or other issues. Somehow the process of putting feelings and thoughts into words brings order and catharsis. Even elementary-school-age children are old enough to be encouraged to keep a journal or to write poems or stories expressing their feelings.

Sharing literature together can also be very therapeutic for grieving children. Several of the references cited in this chapter include lists of age-appropriate books concerning death. As in discussing children's art, it is important to let the children take the lead in determining how much conversation they want in relation to the books they read. The comfort and cuddling that can accompany times of reading together may be as important as what is read.

Two books that can be enjoyed by all ages provide special help in dealing with death. *The Little Prince* by Antoine de Saint-Exupery provides wonderful insights into the nature of love and the meaning of life. In one well-known quotation the little prince, a tiny man from a distant star, prepares to return home. He tells his friend:

> You understand. . . . It is too far. I cannot carry this body with me. It is too heavy . . . but it will be like an old abandoned shell. There is nothing sad about old shells.[30]

And in another classic, *Hope for the Flowers* by Trina Paulus, the metamorphosis from caterpillar to butterfly through the cocoon of apparent death is shown to provide hope and new life.

Support groups have also been found to provide invaluable help throughout the grieving process. Groups for children can be as productive as those for adults, because all people can be comforted by discussing their loss with someone who truly understands. Caregivers who are new to facilitating such groups might find it easiest to begin each meeting with a creative assignment (a picture or poem or clay sculpture) that the children can then share with each other. Or perhaps a relevant (but short) book could be read to the group and then discussed. General questions can also be useful in promoting conversation; for example, What has been hardest for you this week? Children may be slow in becoming comfortable enough to speak out, but group participation can be especially valuable in letting grieving children understand that they are not unique in their pain and that their sorrow will eventually diminish.

Using symbolic and nonsymbolic, verbal and nonverbal language to *commemorate* the life of a loved one is also an excellent tool toward healing. Commemorating the life of a loved one helps a child realize that while the special person will not return, he or she will be remembered; life will go forward but will carry with it memories of the past. As Grollman writes, "The past travels with us and makes us what we are."[31]

Many of the "tools" previously mentioned for healing can also be used for commemorating. Pictures, poems, stories and songs can all be created in remembrance of the loved one. In addition, children may want to plant a tree as a memorial or take flowers to the grave. They may also want mementos or keepsakes that belonged to the deceased, or they might cherish a special photograph. It is also important, even though painful, to keep the memory of the loved one alive by continuing to share memories, both good and not so good, about the deceased. In that way the loved one can be remembered realistically but with love.

But what happens when there is not "good grief," when the pain—instead of being released in positive ways—is, instead, buried deep within? This possible path to adult dysfunction or even psychopathology also must be examined.

96

UNEXPRESSED GRIEF

One of Dr. Grollman's first suggestions for handling unexpressed grief is this:

> Do allow them to release their emotions. Let them call their feelings by the rightful names: I am angry. I am sad. I am hurt. If they wish, they can scream it out. Or put their thoughts into words—in the form of poetry or a story. Or a song. Even a painting. It is not the expression of these legitimate emotions that is harmful, but their suppression.[32]

When children cover up their negative feelings, especially anger and guilt, one result can be lifelong damage to self-esteem. On either the conscious or unconscious level the child comes to believe, "If I have all these bad feelings, I must be a very bad person." And the child can never be convinced otherwise because his or her thoughts are not spoken aloud. Stated another way:

> The blows of life hurt us. But often those who hurt most are silent. The screamers are better off than their silent counterparts. At least they know they are hurt and are feeling their pain. For various reasons, we don't allow ourselves to experience the pain we feel. Often others are to blame.
>
> They don't want to hear about our pain, or it makes them feel uncomfortable about their own failure to scream, or perhaps it just makes them feel awkward. Therefore, the pain ends up being covered with work, alcohol, sex, drugs, depression, compulsive eating, dieting, and the endless list of acting-out behaviors that indicate to alert observers that all is not well. Having failed to scream, they are now screaming through their disorders, addictions, and compulsions. To scream is normal when facing tragic events. Not to scream may reveal the extent to which we are bleeding to death on the inside.[33]

Children, especially adolescents, have ways of acting out buried grief *in addition* to those mentioned above. They may lose interest in or refuse to do schoolwork. They may engage in "fighting and inappropriate risk-taking" or "denial of grief with an accompanying demonstration of hypermaturity." They may withdraw from family and friends as a defense against being hurt again; "unconsciously, children reason it is better to be the abandoner than the abandoned."[34]

Some of these acting-out behaviors may be temporary; others (drug abuse or sexual promiscuity, for example) may have a lifelong impact. One way, in fact, to distinguish between normal and what has been called "complicated" or "pathological" grieving is the duration of the symptoms. The question is not *how* the child is acting, reacting, or overacting, but for *how long*. After an initial period of mourning, children are often able to work themselves back to some degree of productive and near-normal living. It is important to note, however, that the usual period of mourning is actually much longer than many people assume. For example, there are sharp peaks at the three-month and one-year marks after the death—long after many people think the mourners should be "over it."

As Grollman states:

> Of course the daughter is taking her father's death "terribly." Death is a terrible thing for anyone. She has every right to grieve. . . . [However,] danger signals may be present if children continue to:
> - look sad all the time and experience prolonged depression
> - keep up a hectic pace and cannot relax the way they used to
> - not care about how they dress and look
> - seem tired, or unable to sleep, with their health suffering markedly
> - avoid social activities and wish to be alone more and more
> - be indifferent to school and hobbies they once enjoyed
> - experience feelings of worthlessness and self-incrimination
> - rely on drugs and/or alcohol
> - let their moods control them instead of controlling their moods.[35]

When warning signs such as these *continue* or become more serious after a *reasonable* amount of time has passed, it may be that the child is experiencing a clinical depression. Then additional help is needed.

In addition to or in connection with clinical depression, a child may become suicidal or even homicidal, and a compassionate caregiver should not overlook these frightening possibilities.

Differences Between Uncomplicated Grieving and Clinical Depression

	Uncomplicated Grieving	*Clinical Depression*
Loss	Recognizable, current	Often not recognizable
Reactions	Initially intense, then variable	Intense and persistent
Moods	Labile; acute, not prolonged; heightened when thinking of loss	Mood consistently low; prolonged; pervasive pattern
Behavior	Variable: shifts from sharing one's pain to being alone; responds to some invitations; variable restrictions of pleasure	Either completely withdrawn or fear of being alone No enthusiasm for activity Persistent restrictions of pleasure
Anger	Often expressed	Turned inward, not necessarily expressed
Sadness	Periodic weeping and/or crying	Little variability (inhibited or uncontrolled expression)
Cognitions	Preoccupied with loss; confusion	Preoccupied with self; worthlessness; negative sense of self and the future; self-blame; hopelessness
History	Little or no history of depression or other psychiatric illness	Probable history of depression, psychosis, or other psychiatric illness
Sleep disorders	Periodic difficulties	Regular early morning awakening
Imagery	Vivid dreams, capacity for imagery and fantasy	Imagery tends to be self-punitive
Responsiveness	Responds to warmth and assurance	Hopelessness and helplessness limit response

Source: Alicia Cook and Daniel Dworkin, Helping the Bereaved *(Basic Books, 1992), 52.*

Choices such as these would obviously have lifelong impact, but unresolved grief can have other long-term consequences as well. Granger Westberg writes:

> As clergyman in a medical center, where I have worked closely with doctors and their patients for many years, I have slowly become aware of the fact that many of the patients I see are ill because of some unresolved grief situation. . . . I see this so often that I cannot help drawing the conclusion that there is a stronger relationship than we have ever thought between illness and way in which a person handles a great loss. Some of these people who have physical symptoms of distress have stopped at one of the stages in the . . . grief process. Unless someone can help them to work through the emotional problems involved in the stage in which they seem to be fixed, they will remain ill. No amount of medicine will significantly change the situation.[36]

Obviously, long-term emotional problems are at least as likely to occur as physical problems when grieving is not resolved. In the *Manual of Child Psychopathology*, two separate studies "stress the preventative value of accomplishing the 'work of mourning' and the possible ill effects of 'bypassing' the mourning experience." These studies consider that the stoic family member, who may gain applause for not being upset in the face of having lost a loved one, is headed for emotional troubles.[37]

One example of such emotional problems may be an inability to develop or maintain close relationships in adulthood. In studies by psychologist John Bowlby, young children who were separated from their mothers experienced "three successive psychological phases . . . protest, despair, and detachment.[38] Detachment has been discussed previously in examples when a child withdraws from relationships and erects defenses against further relationships/further pain. But the detachment and defenses can become strong enough to inhibit significant relationships throughout life. Daniel Sweeney explains a related phenomenon:

> Attachment disorders are additional ways children may respond to trauma. Attachment is vital for survival, so it is

understandable that threats to attachment are life-and-death issues for children. Children may experience attachment disorders from repeated traumatizing events that prevent a secure attachment from forming or from a single event such as parental abandonment, death of a parent or removal from the home.[39]

Children also may develop long-term relationship difficulties when one parent dies and the remaining parent treats a child as a surrogate spouse—either emotionally (in terms of dependency), physically (by assigning unreasonable responsibility), or, in some cases, sexually. Such interaction effectively robs the child of his or her childhood and may cause tremendous self-esteem and identity problems in addition to relational problems.

As these potential negative outcomes indicate, the reasons for resolving grief through expression rather than burying it through suppression are compelling. And when the potential for lifelong damage to relational skills is included, the significance of helping-healing relationships with compassionate caregivers also becomes obvious. Grief *can* become "good grief" in the presence of love and understanding, and the path to dysfunction and psychopathology *can* be avoided. Two final suggestions remain to be made, however, for those very special people who are willing to do the difficult, painful job of walking with hurting children through their grief—trust God and then trust yourself.

BINDING UP THE BROKENHEARTED
Isaiah 61:1 provides excellent guidance for compassionate caregivers:

> The spirit of the Lord GOD is upon me,
> because the LORD has anointed me;
> he has sent me to bring good news to the oppressed,
> to bind up the brokenhearted.

When God calls people to do a job, God also empowers them for that task. If you feel led to bind up the brokenhearted, especially children who are grieving, the Spirit of the Lord will be upon you to do that work. Hopefully, this chapter has provided you with an increased understanding of the grieving process and some resources to help children as they go through that process. More important than knowledge or skills, however, is a willingness to let God do his work through you. Perhaps the familiar triad— faith, hope, love—can provide you with goals for yourself, for others and for the children with whom you work.

As you have faith in God, God can help you find ways to encourage others also to trust him. What a life-changing experience it can be to learn, especially at an early age, that God's grace is sufficient even in the most painful circumstances. And hope follows naturally after faith. As was stated at the beginning of this chapter, "we know that all things work together for good for those who love God, who are called according to his purpose" (Rom. 8:28). God, in fact, "by the power at work within us is able to accomplish abundantly far more than all we can ask or imagine" (Eph. 3:20).

Faith in God, which is supported by these two promises alone, is certain to produce hope. It is important to remember, however, the familiar words of 1 Corinthians 13:13: "And now faith, hope and love abide, these three; and the greatest of these is love." Your love for the children with whom you work is the greatest gift you give them. It is love that will help to heal them; love that quite possibly can open their eyes to the One who loves them most. In addition, an important avenue of healing for grieving children may be the encouragement to try to pass that love on to others. In the words of Dr. Peale:

> The best of all ways to get your mind off your own troubles is to try to help someone with his. As the old Chinese proverb says, "When I dig another out of trouble, the hole from which I lift him is the place where I bury my own." . . . Carrie Chapman Catt used to have a prescription for curing the blues. It went something like this: "Go to your room; put on your hat; go out and do something for someone. Repeat ten times."[40]

Simply stated, the best thing you can do to "bind up the brokenhearted" is to trust God to use you as a channel for his love and healing. It is also important to remember, however, that God can use you just as you are. Sometimes knowledge and skills take second place to just "being yourself." A wonderful example of this is given in *Roses in December,* written by Marilyn Heavilin, a mother who had lost three children. In one chapter, "The Rose of Hope," Heavilin turns authorship over to her now-grown son, who writes about his memories of being a grieving sibling. These passages are quoted in some detail because they show clearly that sometimes one's best efforts *are* enough—and they provide wonderful insight into grief from a child's perspective:

> I must admit that the family funerals (plural) of my early childhood are somewhat jumbled in my memories. . . . But all the vague images recalled more than thirty years later still crystallize into one very clear thought, evident even then to a five-year-old child: This is an important event, but it is not about me, and no one here has told me where I fit in. In my innocence, I questioned the adults around me. What are we supposed to do now? It had not yet occurred to me that they were probably asking themselves the very same thing. But I persisted in my questions, and someone at last offered an answer, one that I got repeatedly with great conviction and compassion from at least three different adults (not my parents) in at least as many different scenes, "Don't worry. We'll get you ice cream."
>
> Almost two decades later I again found myself dressed in coat and tie, wearing my Sunday best as it were, sitting in the hallway of a mortuary. I was now twenty-three and the last of my brothers, Nathan, lay in state just a few yards away. . . . I could see my own parents making a deliberate effort to keep me involved. We were close to wrapping up the services when my father spoke to me directly, "Your mother and I have got to get out of here. I need you to stay behind and see to it that everything is taken care of." My orders had finally arrived, and I was determined to see them through. However, as I reviewed the scene before me, for all my effort, I couldn't find a single task that had been left unattended. In every case, a courteous professional was doing his job. I eventually rounded up my brother's classmates, piled them into several cars, and we all ended up at Baskin-Robbins

ice cream store. It was smack in the middle of February but I seemed to recall someone mentioning once upon a time that ice cream was therapeutic in these situations.

My eldest son, Nathaniel, is roughly the same age today that I was when I experienced bereavement. These days he is very concerned about his several great-grandparents who have gone on to heaven, as well as his elders who remain here with us. Some nights I find him crying in his bed when he should be sound asleep. So I sit there in the dark with him and we talk and we share our thoughts and our hopes and our fears and our dreams. We talk about recognition because Nathan wants Grandma to be remembered. We talk about rituals and traditions because Nathan wants to know why we do what we do. We talk about reality because Nathan wants to know the truth. We talk about responsibility, because, almost more than anything else, Nathan wants to know what is expected of him. And I tell Nathan every last thing I know. . . . But when the questions just get too tough, or the nights just get too long, or the answers just don't seem to come easily, I promise him with great conviction, "Don't worry, son. We'll get you ice cream." He seems to understand.[41]

Notes

1. James White, *Grieving: Our Path Back to Peace* (Minneapolis, Minn.: Bethany House Publishers, 1997), 83.

2. Phyllis Kilbourn, ed., *Healing the Children of War* (Monrovia, Calif.: MARC Publications, 1995), 1.

3. Granger Westberg, *Good Grief* (Philadelphia: Fortress Press, 1971).

4. Alan Wolfelt, *A Child's View of Grief* (Service Corporation International, 1990), 3.

5. Ibid., 28.

6. Ibid., 33.

7. Ibid., 7.

8. Norman Vincent Peale, *Let Not Your Heart Be Troubled* (Pawling, N.Y.: Foundation for Christian Living, 1997), 17.

9. Theresa Huntley, *Helping Children Grieve* (Minneapolis, Minn.: Augsburg, 1991), 22.

10. Earl Grollman, *Talking About Death* (Boston: Beacon Press, 1990), 39.

11. Ibid., 2.

12. Ibid., 40, 42, 44.

13. Ibid., 43.

14. Elisabeth Kubler-Ross, *Coping with Death and with Dying* (personal audio tapes, 1973).

15. Wolfelt, *A Child's View of Grief,* 9.

16. White, *Grieving,* 37–38.

17. Grollman, *Talking About Death,* 37–38.

18. Wolfelt, *A Child's View of Grief,* 11.

19. White, *Grieving,* 83.

20. Wolfelt, *A Child's View of Grief,* 12.

21. Grollman, *Talking About Death,* 53.

22. Westburg, *Good Grief,* 29–31.

23. Roberta, Temes, *The Empty Place* (Fall Hills, N.J.: Small Horizons, 1992).

24. Grollman, *Talking About Death,* 50–51.

25. Jill Krementz, *How It Feels When a Parent Dies* (New York: Alfred A. Knoff, 1993).

26. Wolfelt, *A Child's View of Grief,* 15.

27. William Worden, quoted in Huntley, *Helping Children Grieve,* 37.

28. H. Norman Wright, *Recovering from the Losses of Life* (Grand Rapids, Mich.: Fleming H. Revell, 1997), 224.

29. For an excellent chapter on the use of play as a method of therapy, see Daniel Sweeney, "Counseling Sexually Exploited Children," in *Sexually Exploited Children: Working to Protect and Heal,* ed. Phyllis Kilbourn and Marjorie McDermid, 109–28 (Monrovia, Calif.: MARC Publications, 1998).

30. Antoine de Saint-Exupery, *The Little Prince* (1943), 87.

31. Ibid., *Talking About Death,* 54.

32. Ibid., 4.

33. Chaplain Robert Hicks, quoted in Wright, *Recovering from the Losses of Life,* 170.

34. Wolfelt, *A Child's View of Grief,* 27, 14.

35. Grollman, *Talking About Death,* 74.

36. Westberg, *Good Grief,* 35.

37. Bejamin B. Wolman, *Manual of Child Psychopathology* (New York: McGraw-Hill, 1972), 199.

38. Ibid., 504.

39. Daniel Sweeney, quoted in Kilbourn and McDermid, *Sexually Exploited Children,* 115.

40. Peale, *Let Not Your Heart Be Troubled,* 17.

41. Marilyn Heavilin, *Roses in December: A Guide to Grieving* (Eugene, Ore.: Harvest House Publishers, 1987), 90–94.

8

Spiritual Nurture for Children Affected by HIV/AIDS

Nancy Huff

Five-year-old Justin sat on his mother's lap and played with the suction dart from a plastic gun. Finally he stuck the suction end on his forehead and announced, "I got AIDS. It hit me just like this." He laughed.

His mother pulled him closer to her chest and asked, "What do you tell people when they ask you why you are sick?"

Justin raised his two hands above his head, touching his two index fingers together, then made a big circle as he brought the two fingers together in his lap. "I only tell friends I have AIDS if they are inside my circle. I don't tell anybody outside my circle. I don't talk outside my circle. That opens a whole big lot of questions if I talk to people outside my circle." His five-year-old mind understood that some people had to know about his illness, and those people were inside his imaginary circle of trusted friends. Those people who didn't have to know were "outside his circle." That's how he categorized whom he talked to and whom he did not. What a beautiful analogy. Isaiah tells us that "God sits enthroned above the circle of the earth." His circle includes all of humanity. He leaves no one out, and there is no one to whom he cannot tell his secrets. He desires that we know the hurts of those around us, like Justin and his mom. His plan is that we reach out and become a part of Justin's circle, that we love him for who he is and accept him and his family as a part of God's wonderful creation.

106

Individuals from a Methodist church, down the road from the little house where he lives, come by to pick Justin up for Sunday school and take him to counseling on Wednesdays. While a lot of churches have extended their hands to the "Justins" in this world, in many towns the church functions on one side of town and the "Justins" live on the other. The two worlds have not become one circle. Does the church, as a whole, care whether Justin grows to become a force for God in this world?

How should the church nurture the ever-growing segment of the world that has been infected by the HIV/AIDS virus? What should our attitude be toward children who die in numbers that increase exponentially each year? What is the heart of God for these children? The problem is so huge, is it even possible to do anything that will help these children? Can Christians make a positive change in the lives of so many who are faced with impending death, and a horrible death at that? How do we implement change?

Children in the throes of AIDS have a kaleidoscope of needs that can be met only by individual attention. Christians can no longer wait for the church as a whole to move into this arena. It must be done by each of us implementing change in attitudes and behaviors so that they reflect a genuine love and concern for hurting children.

Christians can become a force for good in this world. God is a God that looks at the impossible and calls it possible. For any change, God uses individuals. The need here is not just for social change, but for Christians to value the worth of a child and realize that each child has a divine destiny and, given the opportunity, will make a positive contribution to society that will count for eternity. God looks for those who have a parent's heart, who will stand before him in prayer and intercession, and who are willing to take action on behalf of those who are suffering. The challenge is open to everyone. Traditionally, the church has reached out to the poor and hurting, but the onslaught of AIDS in the 1980s and 1990s and the first years of the new century has made the demand for action immediate. If we are to make a difference, the time is now. Are we willing to accept the responsibility of caring for children who are the most rejected segment of society?

PRACTICAL INTERVENTIONS

In the past, globally, Christians have been the most benevolent of all major religions. The reason is because Jesus, by example, taught us to have compassion and to reach out to the poor, sick and needy. Jesus' mission on this earth as prophesied by Isaiah gives a clear picture of what Jesus' attitude would be toward those with HIV/AIDS:

> He shall not judge by what his eyes see,
>   or decide by what his ears hear;
> but with righteousness he shall judge the poor,
>   and decide with equity for the meek of the earth.
>   (Isa. 11:3–4).

Traditionally, the church has reached out to the suffering. Jonathan Kozol, a Jewish author who writes on children's issues, relates his encounter with the churches who minister to the poor in the South Bronx suburb of New York City. South Bronx is home to one of the largest racially segregated concentrations of poor people in the United States. In *Amazing Grace* Kozol writes: "Saddened by the streets, I am repeatedly attracted into churches. I search them out. . . . Meeting these men and women (pastors) is a stirring experience for me. They are among the most unselfish people I have ever known. Many really do see Jesus in the faces of the poorest people whom they serve."[1] This ministry to the poor is so clear that Jesus listed the fact that "the poor have good news brought to them" as one of the signs that he was the Messiah (Matt. 11:4).

The gravity of the fact that millions of people are infected by the AIDS virus calls us to embrace change. New programs that implement intervention, nurture, education, and one-on-one ministry are desperately needed. In the video "In the Arms of the Angels," a documentary about Women and AIDS, the interviewer asks a man what he thinks of the AIDS epidemic in the United States. The short, stocky young man, dressed in a tee shirt and baseball hat, quickly responds that AIDS is a "gay disease" and is punishment from God. Although the commentator never states whether or not this man is a Christian, it is nonetheless the opinion that most AIDS victims believe Christians hold. But AIDS victims should not be judged, especially the children. We are all individuals on a journey through life. Everyone needs love and compassion. Christians should be the first to offer answers to a lost and dying world. True believers, those who follow Jesus with sincerity, will take action—first of all in prayer but also by implementing social programs that minister.

For most Christians the debate is not *whether* we should reach out to the poor but *how* to do it. How do we minister to children who are terminally ill? These children are being ostracized by society, often rejected by their families, and live with pain and fear on a daily basis.

It is difficult to prepare for the death of a loved one. The impact of the death of a child is often overwhelming. What parent wants to outlive his or her children? We want life to give us time to grow old and see our children have grandchildren; we want to come to a place where we lie down and rest, and death becomes the natural progression of life. Since this is not always the case, Christians find themselves addressing the issues of an early death. AIDS stands at everyone's doorstep and can no longer be ignored. It is time for Christians to take an aggressive attitude toward ministry to children with HIV/AIDS.

A SIMPLE VISIT

Truly, it is "a small world, after all." The Christian community can no longer think of AIDS as "someone else's problem." People are infected hourly and need help. We cannot be like the rich man in Luke 16:19–31, who had no compassion on the beggar, Lazarus, who lingered at his doorstep and begged for crumbs from his table.

We are the bearers of good news, and we hold the answers for those who hurt and those who are dying. If Christians do not get involved, then there is no hope for the world. We can no longer wait for the people infected with AIDS to come to us. We must, out of necessity, seek out children and parents who need help. Some organizations already help facilitate outreach to individuals. The parents and children are looking for answers and will find them. The question is, will it be Jesus that they find?

As one man in the last stages of AIDS said, "If I had a choice between not having AIDS and not knowing Jesus, and having AIDS and knowing Jesus, I would take the latter. I know I am going into eternity to meet a loving God, and that is worth anything I must lose in this life. In the fast lifestyle that I lived before I got sick, I don't see that I would have ever taken time to know God."

One AIDS researcher related that she had to deal with her own lack of belief in God when she interviewed 20 women with HIV/AIDS. The women wanted to reconcile themselves with God. Many found a new relationship with God when a Christian came to visit them; some sought out churches that gave them spiritual nurture and acceptance; several found their solace in New Age philosophies.

Preparing for death is one of the most profoundly healing acts of a lifetime. When a parent prepares a child for death, that parent lays a part of his or her heart in eternity, where the call to God and his heaven is always inside the spirit and just a heartbeat away. Facing death for ourselves or for a child forces us to think about God. One social worker described his work with HIV-infected men and their families in Harlem, New York: "Really, it is very beautiful to see what happens to these men, to some of them at least. Once they look into the face of death, some of them begin to live for the first time. Even those who know they are infected and may not have long to live sometimes go through an inner change that brings to mind a kind of 'resurrection.' I have heard men use that word. 'AIDS is my resurrection!' Men who lived in a narcotic cloud for 15 years open their eyes and notice everything. They see the trees and animals and birds! They finally see their children! They learn how to shop and how to cook. Ordinary little things they never knew and never noticed become precious. So, in this way, on the edge of death, they start to live."[2]

Something as simple as a visit to a family during this time of crisis can make a difference for eternity in their lives. There are many organizations already in place that address AIDS issues and provide vehicles for Christians to become involved with people who need help.

SPEAK THE RIGHT WORD

Becky, an eight year old with AIDS, wrote a note about what kinds of things she liked for her friends to ask her. She said, "I like when people ask, 'When are you going to get well?' and say, 'I hope you

110

get well soon.' The things I hate when people say are, 'You'll never get well' and 'Can I catch your illness?'"[3]

Words that blame, hurt and accuse build walls around those who need God's love the most. "I just wish someone would say 'I love you,'" thirteen-year-old Natasha said. "Instead, my friends tease me, and I can't go to school anymore." Natasha's mother now home-schools her in order to shield her from the taunting insults of her classmates. A child with AIDS suffers the effects of rejection from adults and children alike. Children can be especially cruel and unforgiving.

The cry of the heart of the Christian in dealing with those who live in fear and who deal with rejection and pain on a daily basis is found in Isaiah 50:4, "that I may know how to sustain the weary with a word." The ability to say the right thing at the right time is a learned trait. Everyone searches for the right words to say when tragedy strikes. It is usually when we have not come to grips with our own fears of death and dying that we feel awkward around those who are terminally ill. The secret lies in prayer that God will give the right word at the right time. Have in mind what you will say before you make a visit.

There are some words that should be avoided:

- "This is all for a reason."
- "This is because of your sin."
- "Soon you will be at peace."
- "Don't cry."
- "You're going to get better."
- "Just cheer up."
- "Don't think about it."
- "You will get better in a few days."
- "Terminal."
- "Everything is going to be all right."
- "God must have something special in mind for you."

Do say:

- "How do you feel?"
- "How do you (your child) feel about having AIDS?"

111

- "May I pray for you?"
- "I'm so sorry this happened."
- "God loves you."
- "What can I do to help?"
- "Does this make you feel angry?"

ACCEPT

One woman told of calling a friend when she got the devastating test results that affirmed that she and her infant had HIV. "I thought we had been cut off, so I immediately dialed the number again. He said, 'You don't understand. I don't want to have anything to do with you or anyone else who has AIDS.' I was crushed. At that point I had my first taste of the rejection I have suffered over the last two years."

AIDS children long to be accepted. One six-year-old child, Tanya, aptly described her battle with her peers. "I have AIDS and everyone is different than I am. It feels terrible to have AIDS because my tummy hurts a lot and because, if my friends found out, they wouldn't want to play with me. When I told the kids at school I had AIDS, they made fun of me. Now I want to run away from school. I wish I were not an AIDS patient. I wish I didn't have to take medicine." Another child said this prayer, "God, right now I'm very lonely. I have AIDS and am ill, but nobody will get this disease from playing with me. Please God, I need a friend. Love, Natasha." Parents and children alike often reject the child who is "socially unacceptable." Can the church educate people to accept children like Tanya and Natasha? Education on how to accept others is a necessary element in ministry to AIDS children.

LET THE CHILDREN BE "NORMAL"

The desire to be "normal" runs deep in every child. Children will go to great lengths to dress like everyone else, earn only average grades because everyone in their peer group gets C's, and perform dangerous acts because everyone else does. The child who is terminally ill, especially the child with AIDS, also wants to be "normal," to be accepted as a part of school, church and neighborhood. Any hint of being "different" causes anguish with roots of fear and rejection.

Sean, a 16 year old, whose face broke out in acne-like sores, said, "I hate that this disease makes me abnormal. My friends look at me and turn away because I look like a freak. I just want to run home and never go out of my home again—never."

Children with AIDS often do not tell anyone about their bout with the virus because of the ramifications. Often children with AIDS are ostracized, taunted by classmates, or, as one child put it, "they do mean things to us."

Robert, a fifteen year old with AIDS, wrote this definition of normality: "Being normal would be like not having to take medicine every day of your life. Being normal is like not having to miss so much school because of being sick and needing medical treatments. Being normal is not worrying every day about if and when you will get sick and about how people will treat you at that time. I would do anything so that I could be normal."[4]

By loving acceptance the church can make a child feel "normal." One mother relates how her son, Jonathan, has difficulty sitting on the floor because the AIDS medication causes his legs to cramp. Jonathan's friend Molly looks after him. Molly knows that when the time comes to sit in a circle on the floor, Jonathan needs help. She automatically walks to the closet and picks out a blue pillow and brings it to the circle so he can sit more comfortably with the rest of the children. Such a simple act of kindness shows acceptance, love and being "normal." Molly's actions speak volumes. Acts of kindness, especially when performed child to child, carry great weight.

Chances are Molly was taught to be kind and considerate by a loving parent and/or teacher. One of the most caring things a parent or a church can do is to train children to be kind, helpful and considerate. Acts of kindness give backbone to the gospel that is preached from the pulpit. Seldom do those who need the gospel accept it from just sitting in a pew in a church. It is in the classroom, grocery store and Sunday school room where people interact and are accepted that makes the difference.

Children with AIDS can feel normal if they are allowed to play and interact with other children without being singled out. Play groups and classrooms that include HIV-infected children create an atmosphere where all children can feel "normal."

For years, the church has sung the classic hymn "Rescue the Perishing," written in 1869 by Fanny Crosby, a blind American poetess. The words to this song were born out of her work in a New York mission. Our hearts also should cry out: "Rescue the perishing, care for the dying, snatch them in pity from sin and the grave." The church should be the first to welcome those whom society rejects. We should never be just a safe haven for the middle class. "Even if our gospel is veiled, it is veiled to those who are perishing" (2 Cor. 4:3).

HELP A CHILD "DEFUSE"

Put simply, *defusing* means to assist a child to express his or her experiences and feelings. In a more profound setting, it is the process by which a person provides safe interactive assistance in a small group or one on one to help a child express his or her experiences. Defusing can help a child develop coping skills that heal. In small children the defusing process may happen through drawing. In the Kosovo refugee camps in Macedonia, counselors taped the blank side of used McDonald's posters to a fence and supplied the children with tempera paint and paint brushes. The children expressed their grief, hopes and frustration through simple pictures that spoke volumes about their emotional well-being. The same technique has been used with children suffering from other types of tragedies such as AIDS or the loss of a parent. Drawing offers an option for expression but should never be a "required" activity.

Three discussion steps with the child may precede a drawing. First, talk about AIDS in general, then about AIDS in the family and lastly about how AIDS has affected the child personally. Ask open-ended questions or make statements that allow the child to reflect on what has happened:

- "I often wonder . . . "
- "What happens when you have AIDS?"
- "What does AIDS look like?"
- "Dear God, . . . "
- "What is heaven like?"
- "What is it like to have a mom with AIDS?"

- "The hardest thing about all this is . . . "
- "How should people with AIDS be treated?"
- "What are you feeling?"
- "What has changed in your life?"
- "What dreams do you have about AIDS?"

Your questions may produce a theme for a drawing.

Take time to talk and for the child to draw, then follow the process by a quiet reflective time when the child explains what the picture is about and what it means in his or her particular situation. Allow for silence and shyness. Pray for God's wisdom to help you know what to say in response to what the child says and draws.

Remind the child of other troubled times and how God helped in each situation. Psalm 145:4 says,

> One generation shall laud your works to another;
> and shall declare your mighty acts.

Tell Bible stories and give other examples of how God has worked. Children need reference points in their lives to know that God cares and will answer their prayers. Adult Christians who have gone through difficult situations have a lot to share with children.

HELP FINANCIALLY

"I was totally unprepared for the onslaught of bills," one mother said. "There I was, single, with two small children, and one of them with AIDS, and no help other than my small salary. I tried everything anyone told me about, including health food and alternative medicine. Anything someone would suggest, I tried. We saw improvement with eating right, but I didn't have the money to buy all that expensive organic food. The medicine didn't work, and my son died. Then there was all that missed work because of doctor's appointments and lab work. How nice it would have been to have someone, just anyone, help with the financial end of this disease."

AIDS strikes across all economic sectors, but its heaviest financial blows strike those who exist on the lower end of the economic spectrum. Single mothers make up a large portion of those who must deal with a child with AIDS. They can only hope to make their meager paycheck stretch from the first of one month to the next. With the expense of the care of a dying child, which often prohibits the caregiver from working, and the cost of the drugs, the economic impact is staggering. Even parents who have good jobs often find themselves strapped.

Christians are told that "religion that is pure and undefiled before God, the Father, is this: to care for orphans and widows in their distress, and to keep oneself unstained by the world" (James 1:27).

One woman who taught school spoke of the total financial devastation brought on her as a result of her child's bout with AIDS. "If someone had just brought us some fresh fruit, that would have been wonderful. I can't tell you how much it would have meant if someone from the church would have helped us with just a few groceries every now and then. That would have helped a lot. I will never know." She stared out into space. She did not expect the church to pay her medical bills or to pay for her visits to doctors, but a visit from someone with some food may have made the difference.

Fresh vegetables or a casserole are not expensive items in this society, but they could mean a lot to those facing the death of a child with AIDS.

OFFER COMPASSION

How would Jesus have looked at the 30,000 children in our country who have AIDS? Few would argue that he would scoop up children, regardless of disease, and hold them. Can we do less? We should be moved with compassion toward those who are hurting and dying, those who suffer fear and rejection. Since we represent Jesus, we have the ability to reach out to those in need and minister to them.

BE A GOOD LISTENER

A good listener earns the right to ask life-changing questions. People who live in the middle of a life-and-death situation need to talk, whether it's about the vacation they never will have, the dog that needs a bath, or funeral arrangements. The trouble is that not too many people want to listen, especially when AIDS is at the center of the issue.

Most parents of children with AIDS are single parents, often without any moral or financial support from family. The financial woes brought on by a life-threatening disease are enough to throw any one into a tailspin. One mother, Brenda, said: "I remember once wishing that someone would call and ask my son out to get ice cream. He was at home alone day in and day out, and I worked. He needed to get out of the house. He needed to talk with some-one—anyone who would listen. It would have been wonderful. Nobody saw to it that he was okay." She looked out into space and continued: "The church needs to embrace those who are go-ing through a crisis. I think they thought he was strong and didn't need people, but he did."

Merton and Irene Strommen in *Five Cries of Grief* list five ele-ments of healing when a tragedy strikes a family: the cry of pain, the cry of longing, the cry for supportive love, the cry for under-standing and the cry for significance.[5] In each unfolding of the grief process a supportive listener plays a significant part, first in realizing that death is imminent and finally in the recovery pro-cess for the remaining family members. One teenager dying of AIDS said: "Just let me talk. I need to talk of all the birthdays I won't celebrate and all the basketball games I won't be able to play. Then there are all the friends I will never see again. Let me talk so the years will be mine, at least in my memory."

In all those who have children with AIDS and who have AIDS themselves, listening is on the top of the list of what they would like most from those who minister to them. Listening takes time, and time is a precious commodity for those living a fast-paced life with little or no time for their own families, let alone the troubles of someone else. But time goes slowly for those who are isolated and waiting for the next round of medicine or the impending che-motherapy that will make them feel even more ill.

Betsy Burnham, who was diagnosed with terminal cancer, re-lates the story of a woman whom she hardly knew who dropped by to visit her in the hospital. The visitor said: "I don't know you very well. But I know that you must need a friend right now. I don't have anything much to say, but at least I can listen."[6] The woman proved to be an excellent listener throughout the illness.

We need to listen without judgment, without a hidden agenda, not sitting on the edge of our chair, waiting until the person takes a breath so we can insert what *we* consider to be the pertinent Scripture or response. Good listeners earn the right to say words at the right time that will help and heal. Good listeners "says" they care without saying a word.

You don't have to be a close friend of the family to reach out to someone. Lynda, whose three-year-old son, Justin, had AIDS, received a visit at the hospital from a Christian woman she didn't know. "She was absolutely sent by God. I had just walked out of the hospital room because I couldn't stand to see my little boy go downhill so quickly. I was by myself. She didn't tell me much about herself, but she listened to me talk about late night trips to the hospital and how my family had abandoned us, and how we had no money. She listened and held my hand. She gave me her undivided attention for two hours. I knew she was with me. Before she left, she prayed with me. I didn't remember her name until she called me the next week. She knew I needed a friend."

CHILDREN OF THE WORLD

Data for determining the extent of AIDS among children in developing countries is difficult to obtain. One woman described her experience in rural India. "I know I have seen children with AIDS in India, but I have no way to prove it." Janette Wilson, a nurse-practitioner who holds clinics in the remote villages of Northern India, shook her head from side to side and looked at the ground. "We have no doctors, no medicine, and no labs to do blood work and therefore some things like the AIDS virus have gone undetected. The India I have seen is one where the child has no value in the society. If the child cannot work to help the family or produce an income, then, whether that child is healthy or sick, the child is unwanted. There is little nurturing of children. Life is difficult and there is never enough food or money for the family. Each day is just an existence where the strongest survive. For the most part, when a child becomes ill, that child is left to die. It is very sad.

"The villagers have no knowledge about how to care for the sick and, least of all, children who are ill. The government hospitals in the region require people to purchase their own medicine, take it to the hospital with them, and then pay the hospital nurse to give the shot."

Unfortunately, the same may be said of many developing countries. Where the adults do not receive adequate medical help, children receive even less attention.

When a child dies, everyone loses.

A Heritage of Death

The children die, laden and burdened with the death
of those who gave them life,
Only their death comes more heavily and more
swiftly!
And the gnawing teeth of pain pierce their bodies
more relentlessly.
And though the will to live flickers like a starved
weak, little broken flame,
Yet the claws of death sink more deeply and drain
away the very life more greedily.
And death claims the life and steals the heritage of
the God who gave that life.
And the battle continues—
And lost hope falls to the ground and lies buried
within that cradle grave,
And that child who should have become
—the flower of God's love
—the heir of God's promises
—the executor of God's purposes takes all with
him to the grave.
And the enemy laughs![7]

THE LOVE OF IMPERFECT PEOPLE

Those who want to minister often feel inadequate to meet the emotional and physical demands of AIDS victims. However, God gives us the assurance that if we step out in his name, he will help us in our weaknesses. Jesus took the children in his arms and blessed them. What could be a more profound act of love—and yet so simple—as holding a child? One mother whose five-year-old son has AIDS said: "I know someone really cares if they hold Stephen. You would be surprised at how many people, even doctors, never get close to him."

Anne Lamott prays: "God: I wish you could have some permanence, a guarantee or two, the unconditional love we all long for. 'It would be such skin off your nose?' I demand of God. I never get an answer. But in the meantime I have learned that most of the time, all you have is the moment, and the imperfect love of people."[8]

Notes

1. Jonathan Kozol, *Amazing Grace: The Lives of Children and the Conscience of a Nation* (New York: Crown Publishers, 1995), 78.

2. Ibid., 200.

3. Robert Coles, *Be a Friend: Children with HIV Speak*, (Morton Grove, Ill.: Albert Whitman and Company, 1994), 39.

4. Ibid., 18.

5. Merton and Irene Stommen, *Five Cries of Grief* (Minneapolis, Minn.: Augsburg Fortress Press, 1996).

6. Betsy Burnham, *When Your Friend Is Dying* (Grand Rapids, Mich.: Chosen Books, 1982), 25.

7. Patricia Morgan, *Tell Me Again: The Cry of the Children* (Shippensburg, Pa.: Destiny Image Publishers, 1996), 5.

8. Ann Lamott, *Traveling Mercies: Some Thoughts on Faith* (New York: Pantheon Book, 1999), 168.

PART IV

Strategies for Compassionate Action

9

Orphans: Our Children, Our Responsibility

Susie Howe

What does it feel like to be Sakhile, a 10 year old living in Zimbabwe? Her mother recently died of AIDS. Her father had already died of the same disease. Her country is being ravaged by the AIDS pandemic. Over a quarter of Zimbabwe's 5.5 million adults are HIV infected. The government estimates that in two years time, 2,400 Zimbabweans a week will be dying of AIDS.[1]

AIDS is already devastating the lives of hundreds of thousands of children like Sakhile in Zimbabwe, and millions of children worldwide are experiencing the same overwhelming sense of loss and desolation as they lose their parents to this dispassionate and relentless disease.

No one knows exactly how many children have been orphaned by AIDS worldwide, but a USAIDS publication estimates that close to 42 million children will be orphaned by 2010 in the 23 most affected countries worldwide.[2] AIDS is threatening the lives, development and future of the world's children such as never before.

In this chapter we will be confronted with the truth that the church of Jesus Christ has a mandate from God to lead the way in actively demonstrating his love and compassion to his most vulnerable little ones. We will refer to the experiences of The Bethany Project based in Zvishavane, Zimbabwe, a Christ-centered program that mobilizes the church and whole communities to care compassionately for orphaned children.

JESUS: OUR ROLE MODEL

Time and time again throughout the Gospels, Jesus demonstrated compassion in his robust, practical response to the problems of others. He was empathetic in the way he entered into the world of others and was unconditionally "there" for them. Not only did he stand with them in their predicament, but he responded with appropriate, practical action.

How can we enter into the world of orphan children and stand with them in a way that empowers and strengthens them? To do this effectively, we need to understand some of the difficulties that children who have been orphaned as a result of AIDS encounter. We also need to understand the root cause of those problems.

THE IMPACT OF AIDS ON COMMUNITIES

The AIDS epidemic is severely destabilizing communities where there is a high incidence of HIV. High morbidity and mortality rates affect the economy, agriculture, industry, the labor force, education and every area of community life. As increasing numbers of young adults die, there are fewer caregivers available to provide nurture for orphaned children.

As the young adult population is decimated by AIDS, communities experience a drain on the skills and manpower necessary to develop the community and to impart to its children and youth vital skills and knowledge regarding culture, traditions, social norms and values. Not only does AIDS threaten the survival of vulnerable children, but it also threatens the survival of whole communities. Without energetic and sustained holistic support along with appropriate interventions, we must ask ourselves what the future holds for these children and their communities:

> Not only do these children deserve our humanitarian concern, but the potential social impact of their presence in large numbers demands our immediate attention. The presence of large numbers of under-educated, impoverished, and less-than-healthy children in under-developed social structures may have negative effects on social organizations and societal stability.[3]

THE IMPACT OF AIDS ON CHILDREN

Children suffer unimaginable trauma and psychological pain as they witness the prolonged suffering and eventual death of first one parent, and then the other. They may well be the ones who have to nurse their dying parents while also trying to care for younger siblings. It is by no means unusual for one of the siblings to be dying of AIDS as well. Just because a parent is HIV positive does not mean that the children are necessarily HIV positive. However, about one in three babies born to HIV-positive women are also HIV positive. Two young brothers under 10 years of age who we cared for through the Bethany Project experienced the deaths of their parents, both their grandparents, an aunt and an uncle in the space of four years.

Children who have become the main caregivers are robbed of their childhood as they shoulder burdens that would daunt the average adult. To make matters worse, the stigma and fear that still surrounds AIDS mean that they are unable to confide in others. Secrecy stops them from being able to seek the support that they so badly need. Social isolation may increase their sense of grief and loss.

Further, there is an increasing number of child-headed households where children as young as 10 years of age are trying to look after their siblings with little or no adult supervision. These children are particularly vulnerable and at risk of abuse and exploitation. Volunteers trained by The Bethany Project once found a 12-year-old boy unsuccessfully trying to re-thatch the dilapidated roof of the hut where he lived with his two sisters who were both under 8 years of age. His parents had died the year before; he had assumed the role of "man of the house" with virtually no adult help or assistance.

Orphaned adolescents are forced to navigate their way through this particularly challenging period of their lives without the counsel and support of their parents. Their fragmented education and lack of skills renders them extremely vulnerable economically. They may have many siblings to support without the means to do so. Without holistic support and committed caregivers to provide long-term care, the future for these orphaned children is bleak. It is a frightening reality that the next generation of HIV-infected young adults will have no mothers to care for them when *they* are sick and dying. They also will have no grandparents to act as caregivers to *their* children. It is therefore vital that the church of Jesus Christ be on the front line in giving compassionate care to the world's orphans and in leading the way in AIDS prevention.

COMPASSIONATE CARE OF ORPHANS

"What can we do without money—we are poor ourselves."
"There are too many children to care for."
"It's the government's responsibility to care for these children."
"They should be placed in an orphanage."

These were some of the responses we heard when we first challenged churches and communities to care for their orphans at Bethany Project workshops. Undoubtedly the task of caring for large numbers of needy children is daunting; it is sometimes difficult to know where to start. First and foremost, however, the mandate to care for orphaned children is one that comes from God himself. He is the one who will enable and equip us to make a difference in their lives.

> Seek justice,
>   rescue the oppressed,
> defend the orphan
>   plead for the widow. (Isa. 1:17)

Again and again God exhorts his people to protect orphans and widows. We cannot walk away from our responsibility to help care for these children. There are simply too many orphans to even consider trying to accommodate them in orphanages. The sheer economics involved render this an unviable option, quite apart from the fact that while there are many excellent children's homes in existence, institutional care can be stigmatizing. Also, it can never meet the needs of a child as effectively as raising that child within a loving family context. While governments should undoubtedly support initiatives to care for children at risk and should focus on the prevention of AIDS, the reality is that most orphans and people living with AIDS are to be found in some of the world's poorest nations, where debt and corruption cripple any meaningful government interventions.

So what is the answer? Or perhaps, *Who* is the answer? To put it bluntly, we are. We are God's answer to meeting the needs of the world's orphaned children and to giving them hope for the future. We can begin to do so in myriad different ways.

COMMUNITY-BASED ORPHAN CARE

For the past five years The Bethany Project in Zvishavane has been training whole communities to care for their orphans. Local churches and Christians are encouraged to lead the way in giving practical love and care to the destitute orphan families in their midst and in developing their communities in order to increase their capacity to care for these families. They are encouraged to discuss the problems that orphans face and then to think of practical ways to address those problems, using just their hands, their feet and their hearts, and the resources that they have readily available within their local community. The churches and communities are then encouraged to put these ideas into practice.

Volunteers visit the most destitute orphan families in their communities to give practical help, care and loving support. The help they give requires no particular qualifications other than a real heart of love and concern for the children. Basically, they do the sort of things that any caring mother or father would do for their children. They fetch firewood and water, help to mend broken-down homesteads, plow fields, plant and cultivate maize, teach the children practical skills, pray and share the Scriptures, start income-generating projects (such as peanut-butter making) in order to raise funds to send the children back to school, mend the children's clothing, cook for them, share food with them and generally do whatever is within their capacity to do to improve the quality of life for the children.

They spend time listening to the children's fears and concerns, help them with their homework, and teach them about the skills and traditions that the children will need to integrate into their communities. They also teach them biblical values and, more important, strive to act as good role models so the children can witness those values practiced in everyday life. The volunteers speak

127

up on behalf of the children when necessary. It has been heart-warming to see just how far the volunteers will go to help a child or a child's grandparents.

A small act of kindness can make a big difference to elderly grandparents who are struggling to raise their orphaned grand-children under very difficult circumstances. It makes them realize that they are not abandoned or forgotten; it also encourages them to carry on. In this way nearly 6,000 orphans and children at risk are now being cared for in the Zvishavane district. The attitude of the communities have changed from indifference toward the plight of the children to active concern. The rights of the child are begin-ning to be recognized. Communities are more prepared to speak out against the abuse of those rights. Child molesters are more frequently reported, and unreasonable child labor is less accepted than before. Best of all, children who were once malnourished, unschooled and neglected are now back at school and able to rough and tumble with their friends!

Undoubtedly there are difficulties and frustrations along with a long way to go, but now there is hope where previously there was despair. The churches and communities are realizing that the power to change is within their hands and that with God's help, their own lives can be improved.

When the local church woke up to the challenge of caring for its orphans, life changed dramatically for Peter. The pastor's wife led a small team of women to visit children like Peter, doing all they could to give them loving care and support.

Six-year-old Peter was sick with AIDS and TB. His 75–year-old grandmother was doing her best to care for him and his three broth-ers and sisters, but she too was sick with TB, had a broken arm and was unable to plow or adequately care for the children.

When the volunteers first visited Peter and his grandmother they found him lying listlessly on the floor, in a corner that also housed a pool of muddy rainwater. This was the family's one and only hut. The roof had fallen in; because it was the rainy season, the hut was awash. Peter was seriously sick and emaciated, and his grandmother was no better. The other children scavenged to survive as best they could.

The pastor's wife and her dedicated team mobilized the local villagers, and together they built Peter and his family a new bedroom hut. They also mended the roof and repaired the floor on the old one so it could serve as the kitchen. They plowed, planted and cultivated a field. Until harvest, they gave the family maize from their own granaries and gifts of vegetables and peanut butter.

Peter's younger sister was sent to school, and the pastor's wife regularly took Peter to the clinic. As she washed and dressed him, she told him stories about Jesus and his love for Peter. She prayed with him and his grandmother and often had them stay in her own home.

A year later Peter died at home in the arms of his grandmother. There was enormous comfort knowing that during the last year of his life he had been touched with the hands and love of Jesus through the loving care and commitment of the volunteers. His grandmother, brothers and sisters still receive that same support.

As Christians we have a very real responsibility to reflect the love and values of Jesus Christ in the way we care for orphans and other children at risk. It costs nothing to pray with children or to listen to their worries. It costs nothing to mend their clothing or to teach them a simple skill. It costs nothing to pray and intercede for them. Nothing, that is, but our time and commitment. This commitment has to be a long-term one, partly because it needs to be sustained throughout their childhood and teenage years and partly because erratic commitment can further traumatize a child who has already experienced loss and instability.

There are many ways that we can show compassionate care for orphans. Some of us will be called to support orphan-care programs with prayer, finances, training skills and material assistance. Some of us may be called to volunteer our time to visit an orphan family on a regular basis to give the sort of practical care described in these pages. Others will be called by God to open their hearts and homes to an orphaned child. Others will be asked to campaign for the rights of orphans and people living with AIDS—to be a voice for the voiceless. Although this chapter has focused on orphans living in an African nation, AIDS affects every nation and continent in the world. The culture and social circumstances may differ, but the problems that orphans face, such as grief and confusion over the loss of their parents, stigmatization and increased vulnerability, remain universal. Nations such as America, Romania, Brazil, Russia, India and the UK all have children who are struggling to live with the consequences of AIDS. It may be that there are children and families on our own doorstep who are in need of our loving support, or it may be that we and our church are being called to support an overseas orphan project. As Christians, involving ourselves in the compassionate care of orphans is not an option. It is a mandate from God, and it is to God that we are accountable for our response. Caring for his children is infinitely rewarding. As we invest in their lives, we will experience the joy of seeing God's healing and restoration taking place, ultimately making them into the men and women that God created them to be.

I well remember the joy of seeing 12–year-old Celia smile for the first time. Her parents had died two years previously, and she had become withdrawn, unsmiling and uncommunicative. As her volunteer "aunty" began to visit her on a daily basis, giving her unconditional love, Celia started to change. Her schoolteacher reported that she was starting to participate in class and, as a result, was getting higher marks. Celia would turn up at the home of the volunteer, simply to sit and sew with her in silence. It was a great day for us all when Celia started to join in the games of other children. The day she actually burst out laughing was a great day indeed. She is now a warm and loving child who is as mischievous as the best of children!

No matter what their race, color, or background, these children are *our* children and *our* responsibility. Let us take time to ask God what our individual response to them should be.

Notes

1. "AIDS Epidemic Update," UNAIDS Joint United Nations Programme on HIV/AIDS (December 1998).

2. J. Hunter and S. Williamson, "Children On The Brink: Strategies to Support Children Isolated by HIV/AIDS (Washington, D.C.: USAIDS, 1997).

3. Ibid.

10

Special Concerns
in HIV/AIDS Interventions

Phyllis Kilbourn

"I was hungry and you gave me food,
I was thirsty and you gave me something to drink,
I was a stranger and you welcomed me,
I was naked and you gave me clothing,
I was sick and you took care of me,
I was in prison and you visited me."

"Lord, when was it that we . . . ?"

"Truly I tell you, just as you did it to one of the least of these who
are members of my family, you did it to me."
                                                           —Matthew 25:35–40

The previous chapters have discussed at length the heartaches
and suffering of children affected by HIV/AIDS, suffering
that has been caused not only by physical pain, but also by tremendous multiple losses, separation, bereavement, isolation,
stigma and discrimination. We have also seen how the epidemic
has grossly affected the economic and social fabric of communities at every level, resulting in a rapidly increasing number of orphans and street children.

While there may not be a medical cure for the physical effects
of AIDS, compassionate care can bring hope and emotional and
spiritual healing to those who are so often neglected or left to survive on their own. Christian caregivers have a vital role to play in

131

planning and implementing compassionate, sustainable, preventive and intervention measures. These measures must include a supportive environment; these children have enormous needs for stability and continuity at home, school, church and in the community. Providing measures that offer children an abundance of healing doses of love, care, acceptance and attention, along with emotional and spiritual support, constitutes a compassionate response.

INTERVENTION CONCERNS

Before planning prevention and intervention programs, one needs to be aware of the unique issues begging to be addressed. This section introduces some vital issues: poverty, special family concerns, trauma, protection of children's rights, ethical issues, early treatment of HIV-positive pregnant women and non-infected children.

Poverty

It must be remembered that AIDS is an economic issue as well as a health issue. AIDS has been described as a poverty-seeking missile. HIV infection not only thrives in impoverished environments, but also the disease itself is a potent cause of poverty. Poverty hastens deaths among AIDS sufferers. And in places such as southern Africa, the sheer number of AIDS deaths aggravates the poverty of those who survive.

The pain AIDS inflicts is economic as well as physical, since it deprives the person of his or her ability to work in the latter stages of the disease, condemning the family to heightened poverty. Loss of work coupled with the high cost of seeking medical treatment and funeral expenses leaves few resources for the children's survival. Thus they are forced to enter the labor market at a very early age.

Clearly, the chain of intervention for AIDS orphans must include a link to address the economic impoverishment of the family and the community. In particular, assistance must be provided for those who are willing, or of necessity are forced, to become caregivers—including children, who often have to assume responsibilities as head of household at a very early age.

Susan Hunter and John Williamson caution us against singling out for assistance those children whose parents have died with AIDS, as it stigmatizes the intended beneficiaries. The needs of individual children are not necessarily greater than those of children orphaned by other causes or vulnerable for other reasons, and the problems may begin long before their parents become ill or die from AIDS. Because of increased economic stress on households many children who are not orphans will also experience problems. Therefore, they advise:

> Interventions should be targeted in two stages. They should be directed to the communities where the impact of HIV/AIDS is greatest and where it significantly affects the ability of families to meet their children's needs. Within these communities, assistance should be targeted to the children and families identified by residents as the most vulnerable (without making HIV/AIDS a criterion).[1]

Special Family Concerns

Because problems caused by HIV/AIDS are shared by all members of a household, the focus of care for AIDS patients must be on the family. Poverty, a lack of access to institutional care, personal preference and cultural norms allow few opportunities for care outside family structures. Changes in family composition and increased poverty also limit the ability of many families to provide needed care for sick family members.

Families usually cannot afford even basic medicines to treat opportunistic infections or to make afflicted family members comfortable. The demands of caring for sick family members may lead caregivers to neglect their own needs or those of others in the household. Caregivers can benefit from the support of members of their extended families or communities and from counseling to address the stigma, isolation and uncertainty they feel about the future.

Children, family situations and needs for intervention vary. The problems of children affected by HIV/AIDS, however, begin long before their parents die and extend beyond their individual households to affect relatives, neighbors and whole communities.

Intervention planning, therefore, must target communities and all children affected by HIV/AIDS, not just those whose parents have been infected with HIV or have died of AIDS. With an HIV-infected child, families may need help providing the child with adequate care, including emotional support and good nutrition. Caregivers may also need help to take on an advocacy role for these children, promoting nondiscrimination policies and programs so that affected children are treated with dignity. Our overall goal should be to offer the children an opportunity to have as normal a childhood as possible. We also have to think of their future—their survival (food, clothing and shelter) and protecting their legal rights to their parents' property.

Trauma

Living through the stigma of having a parent with "the disease" and witnessing his or her slow, often agonizing death causes great emotional stress and trauma. The deprivation of maternal care results in varying degrees of acute anxiety and an excessive need for love. Forming and maintaining emotional ties with caring adults is crucial to a child's emotional well-being.

For those afflicted with HIV/AIDS, the trauma is never ending. Fears, stigma, losses, uncertainties and despair for a meaningful future deeply affects their emotional well-being. Their health-related traumas are compounded by the deaths of parents, siblings and friends.

For most children, stigmatization, dropping out of school, changing friends, carrying an increased workload, suffering discrimination and social isolation increase their stress. Difficult relationships with new caregivers can also be a significant stress factor. Stress can cause children to become depressed, reducing their ability to cope with the new and ever-growing pressures.

Bereavement counseling and strengthening of coping skills are needed for traumatized children to move beyond their grief issues and gain a new perspective on their situations. Children's psychological needs are best met when they are allowed to remain integral members of their communities, finding security in familiar structures and community networks.

Protection of Children's Rights

Measures are needed to safeguard children's legal rights, especially to ownership of the parental home and land. Without a will or legal document, land-hungry relatives quickly bilk the children out of their rightful inheritance. Also, in informal fostering relationships—common because legal work is time consuming—orphans enjoy fewer legal rights than other children. Fostering adults often claim the children's property as theirs since they have assumed care for the children. Keeping land within a family is often a very important cultural value and tradition. Land ownership also provides a sense of tribal and community identity.

Ethical Issues

Caregivers need to consider the ethical issues they will confront in planning their strategies and programs. UNAID advocates considering the following ethical issues that underpin work with children and young people affected by AIDS. In light of the issues that will be encountered, caregivers should write a similar set of guidelines based on their convictions. UNAID's convictions rest on the premise that all children's programs should promote the rights and interests of children and young people while restoring or maintaining their dignity.

1. The best interests of the child should always be put first.
2. Children's right to decide for themselves should be respected at all times and care taken to ensure that the children understand the implications of their participation and know that they can refuse to participate.
3. Children's rights to confidentiality and freedom from discrimination should not be compromised by participating.
4. Children should participate in an environment where they feel safe with their own peers so that do not feel threatened, frightened or used.
5. Children should not be portrayed in a negative and disadvantaged way.
6. Children should not be exploited for commercial, medical or research purposes.

7. Children and parents/carers should be involved in negotiating policies to ensure that they are child-centered.[2]

Early Treatment of HIV-positive Pregnant Women

The fastest growing group of children with HIV infection and related illnesses is infants who are being infected through perinatal, mother-to-child transmission. This transmission of HIV to infants can be prevented by providing antiretroviral drugs to HIV-positive pregnant women. The antiretroviral drug ATZ was found effective in field trials in Thailand and is significantly cheaper than other treatments. UNICEF predicts this drug will help fuel a major expansion of the war against AIDS in the developing world.

Non-infected Children

We must not forget the needs of children who are not HIV infected yet have HIV-infected parents or siblings. They, too, need psychological and emotional support in order to

- understand what is happening to the person with AIDS.
- deal with their own feelings (worry, fear, anger, sadness, confusion).
- know what to tell their friends and other people.
- deal with the possibility of losing a very important person (parent, sibling).
- know they are loved and that they will be cared for and not left alone. (One of the greatest fears of non-infected as well as infected children of HIV-infected parents is that they will be left alone.)
- deal with the stresses that the reality of AIDS brings.

PREVENTION STRATEGIES

Programs on awareness, knowledge and advocacy are needed if we are to educate the public and bring a halt to the spread of this deadly disease. Misconceptions of the cause of AIDS abound. Curses, charms and the evil eye provide fertile ground for speculating on the causes, especially among animistic African peoples and cultural Hindus. It is thought that if a person dies of AIDS, it is the result of a curse put on him or her by a family member, an enemy, fetish priest or dead ancestor.

"The way some people think of it, if AIDS were caused by sexual promiscuity, everybody would be dead, so that can't be it," explains a Zambian pastor. "For these people, their efforts at prevention are limited to sacrifices and appeasement of spirits. They simply look for supernatural causes and solutions."[3]

An area in prevention is alerting parents to the necessity of talking about their illness and its consequences for the children and planning culturally relevant sex education programs.

Advocacy

Caregivers should encourage governments to provide legal status through which children's advocacy can be voiced. Governments need to mobilize people at the grass-roots levels so initiatives can be participatory rather than government directives. The community should have a clear sense of ownership.

As caregivers become engaged in working with children affected by HIV/AIDS, they will develop an awareness and understanding of the children's community, along with its problems and resources. The most successful methods for advocacy will also become evident. Advocacy can mean raising a voice on behalf of children to:

- change community attitudes toward families with HIV/AIDS and thus reduce the discrimination that hinders their normal living patterns.
- create a greater public awareness and understanding of the families' problems, especially the children who are infected with HIV and the orphans.
- tap into local sources of funding and resources to meet the children's basic needs such as nutritional food, medical care, shelter, education and parental support.
- identify obstacles preventing change and planning strategies to remove those obstacles.
- rally support for families whose health status prevents them from working and caring for the needs of their family.

- influence government policy and practice regarding children's need for protection, safety and general well-being.
- protest the unfair advantage taken of children who are forced to earn a living for their parents and/or siblings.

Mass media channels are powerful tools for advocacy. Radio, TV, posters, newspaper, drama, songs, rallies, boycotts and community forums are a few examples.

Awareness Programs

Whether motivated by fear, embarrassment or ignorance, many people refuse to talk about or acknowledge HIV/AIDS. Cultural beliefs and values also prevent some from talking freely about these issues. Japan, for example, is a group-oriented society, and shame is an important factor. HIV/AIDS is shameful not only for them but also for their family. Few Japanese patients reveal that they are infected.

Such silence has had deadly consequences for millions who have not been reached with vital messages of awareness and prevention. Only when people are willing to discuss HIV/AIDS, sexuality and drug use openly will we begin to remove the stigma that surrounds this disease. Then we can promote powerful national and local prevention efforts that will effectively curb the spread of this deadly epidemic.

To end the silence, caregivers and community educators need to:

1. Listen to others as they speak about HIV and about their fears and misconceptions. Engage them in culturally relevant conversation about issues such as sexuality, drug use and the behaviors that put them at risk for HIV/AIDS.

2. Learn from one another: the young from adults, adults from youth, youth from each other, HIV negative from HIV positive. Help others learn about respect, support and protection from HIV.

3. Live in a manner that serves as a model of safe behaviors that prevent the spread of HIV.[4]

Preparing Children for Independent Living

Most parents are secretive about having AIDS, leaving the children uninformed. They may want to hide their HIV status to preserve the dignity and self-respect of the family, protect their children from social ostracization or prevent discrimination in housing, employment and medical care. Parents also may refuse to tell their children about their HIV status out of shame, self-hatred, fear of rejection or concern that the children will insist on giving up their own life to care for the parent.

When parents are diagnosed with HIV, however, they should be encouraged to demonstrate courage in informing the children and to begin preparing them for future responsibilities. Disclosing this information also facilitates the children's anticipatory grief process, better preparing them for the time the parent does die.

Caregivers can help parents prepare their children for life after their deaths. Parents agonize over the thought of leaving their children without their guidance; advance preparation will give them peace of mind. Some steps caregivers can guide parents into taking on behalf of their children include:

- finding another family or person who can care for and shelter them. This is where the church can play a major role.
- making a will. This is very important to protect the property normally grabbed by next of kin, leaving children with nothing.
- avoiding debt burdens because of their illness. This should also include the planning of a simple funeral to hold down costs of funeral debt.
- passing on skills and knowledge to children so they can become economically independent. It also could include seeing that the children are apprenticed to a community worker who can train them in a marketable, income-generating skill.
- teaching the children to take measures to protect themselves and others while caring for the sick. They need to know they can become infected from contaminated body fluids, especially when they are cleaning or dressing open wounds or cuts.

Caregivers can also assist the church and community in discovering meaningful ways to become involved with the children's needs and problems. The church can play an active and essential role in fulfilling missing family functions, such as

- maintaining and nurturing relationships before and after the parents have died. Loneliness and isolation will intensify the children's problems.
- planning and working with the children in guiding their future. Children should be involved in the planning.
- providing opportunities for children to continue their education.
- addressing children's social and sexual development needs through family-based care.

Sex Education

Being vulnerable and powerless, the girl child is especially at risk of HIV/AIDS. Street life, sex tourism, forced child labor, serving as child soldiers and most other forms of exploitation involve sexual abuse. Early marriage also places the girl child at risk. Children's tissues are thin and can easily tear during sexual intercourse, allowing the virus to enter the blood stream.

If a girl cannot be moved away from the abuse and into a safe environment, she must be given the opportunity to protect herself. This protection must include the availability of condoms and appropriate education on keeping safe. Girls also need to be provided with alternatives. If, for example, prostitution is the only way young girls have for earning an income, job skills will have to be taught to enable them to gain employment in safe jobs.

Girls also should be taught how to identify and approach "safe persons" for counseling and help when needed. These safe persons (such as dedicated caregivers, teachers, social workers or counselors) can be a sanctuary for vulnerable girls. They also can provide them with the needed sex education.

Community education is vital to make families and communities aware of how exploitation and early marriage place their children at risk. Childhood is a special time God has planned for children to be carefree and protected, enabling them to grow and develop according to normal patterns. Valuing a safe childhood for girl children must be embraced at all levels of society, including the legal systems. The importance of protecting the girl child cannot be overemphasized.

Primary HIV prevention focuses on keeping people from becoming infected with HIV and on helping those who are HIV positive develop skills for reducing the risk of infecting others. Thus sex education starting at an early age is vital. Children and youth must be taught that a chaste lifestyle is the first line of defense against contracting HIV infection.

If HIV prevention fails among the young, we will have to face the staggering human and economic costs of vast numbers of new AIDS cases. Prevention is the first and most powerful strategy we have to protect caregivers and others from becoming infected with HIV. Only when everyone has the facts, especially concerning sexual and drug transmission, can we go ahead with effective prevention programs.

When everyone feels free to discuss HIV/AIDS openly, caregivers can confront the misinformation, fears and discrimination that are now perpetuating the spread of the disease. Such a change in attitude must begin at the community level—in the church and other local community structures.

INTERVENTION STRATEGIES

Because the pandemic and its consequences will be with us for generations, individuals, families and communities must be prepared to cope with HIV and AIDS over the long term. With millions affected and limited available resources, programs to prevent, control and mitigate the effects of HIV/AIDS will require active involvement of the churches in their communities. Intervention programs should be designed that:

- minimize children's psychological and emotional trauma
- keep orphans as integral members of their community.
- include an understanding of needs at the family and community levels.
- address basic material needs.
- provide opportunities for education, vocational training and employment creation for adolescents.

141

For intervention strategies to be effective in helping children, families and communities affected by HIV/AIDs, they must:

1. strengthen the capacity of families to cope with their problems.
2. stimulate and strengthen community-based responses.
3. ensure that governments protect the most vulnerable children and provide essential services.
4. build the capacities of children to support themselves.
5. create an enabling environment for affected children and families.
6. monitor the impact of HIV/AIDS on children and families.[5]

The following community and church-based programs for those affected by HIV/AIDS demonstrates some of these intervention principles.

Community-based Care

Community-based care programs are viewed as the most effective treatment programs for children with AIDS. A community-based program allows children to remain in their own communities and family members to remain together; this facilitates greater normalization in the children's upbringing. These programs are also more economically viable. Owned and run by the community, the sustainability of a program is enhanced.

Orphan-care and attending to the needs of children suffering from HIV/AIDS also are tasks that affect whole communities. Poor families already struggling to care for their own children have an even greater financial burden when orphans are added into the extended family or a sick child needs medical attention. Many times when a father dies, mothers are left without a financial base to care for the children. Or parents' deaths turn older people into primary caregivers while at the same time depriving them of support from their adult children. One elderly Zambian grandmother, having buried all five of her children, now struggles to take care of the 25 grandchildren left behind.

In light of the magnitude of the task of caring for these orphans and children afflicted with HIV/AIDS, many view community-based care as the most effective method of intervention. The needs of the families and communities of those affected by HIV/AIDS must be addressed along with the children's needs. Zimbabwe provides a good case study for community-based care. Here children remain in their communities, have child-headed homes and rely on a supportive community that backs their efforts.

Zimbabwe Case Study

AIDS has been spreading rapidly in Zimbabwe, as in other sub-Saharan African countries. Recognizing a need for a legal framework for the provision of care for orphans within the country, the Department of Social Welfare helped develop a National Orphans Care Policy that emphasized the need for children to be raised within their own communities. Their valuing of community support is evident by their belief that it is preferable for orphans to be cared for in community-supported, child-headed households rather than by being fostered, adopted or cared for in any type of institution.

The Family AIDS Caring Trust (FACT), also firm in its conviction that communities have a key role in supporting their own orphans, are concerned that interventions develop and strengthen existing coping mechanisms rather than undermine them. If families, for example, look directly to an NGO for support rather than to their community, it is likely that coping strategies are being undermined. FACT feels the effectiveness of community programs can be evaluated through a community's ability to:

- provide human resources to monitor orphan families through programs of regular visiting.
- more accurately prioritize children in most need.
- provide practical support to the children, such as farming, repairing homes.
- make accessible to the children existing educational and health facilities.
- provide in-home services for terminally ill children.[6]

Because communities often are poor, resources need to be channeled into community initiatives and away from the development of additional institutional care facilities or residential homes.

143

Church-based Response

With the diagnosis of HIV/AIDS comes much shock, grief and fear. To protect and provide for the needs of the children whose parents are affected by AIDS, we must provide ongoing support for their families. Only when families receive the needed emotional, spiritual and practical support can they give time to helping their children through the crisis.

For many individuals and families, a flood of questions and unknowns immediately surfaces when they learn of their AIDS. Who will care for me when I am no longer able to walk without assistance? Who will care for the children? How can we keep up with the cooking, laundry and yard work that need to be done? Will there be anyone who could help with my care as I become weaker and my caregivers become exhausted? Will I be able to stay in my own home surrounded by my family when I am dying? Will I die alone?

AIDS Interfaith Ministries (AIM), located in Louisville, Kentucky, is attempting to answer these questions and similar concerns by offering to match individuals and families touched by HIV and AIDS with "care teams" made up of volunteers. The AIDS Care Teams Program is one of several ministries of AIM of Kentuckiana. Founded in 1990, AIM of Kentuckiana is a group of clergy, laity, community professional and volunteers representing all faith perspectives committed to ministry and education related to the HIV/AIDS pandemic. AIM of Kentuckiana's purpose is to develop spiritual, emotional and ethical resources for persons both infected and affected by HIV/AIDS. AIM compiles and evaluates the availability of culturally and religiously sensitive HIV/AIDS prevention. The organization works to raise awareness of the global aspects of HIV/AIDS and promotes a compassionate interfaith response to AIDS.

Teams of no fewer than six people provide gap-filling services not covered by other AIDS service providers or reimbursable by medical insurance, services that are valuable in helping to keep individuals at home and families together. Care teams, people of faith with a variety of skills and talents, rely upon one another for support in caring for an individual or family living with HIV rather than expecting one individual to carry the weight and responsibility of providing volunteer services.

AIM of Kentuckiana Care Teams Program augments and enhances both the formal and informal caregiving of individuals and families living with HIV and AIDS by providing services such as the following:

- transportation and accompaniment to health and legal appointments.
- shopping.
- light housekeeping.
- meal preparation.
- minor home repairs.
- car repairs.
- friendly visiting.
- light yard work.

Care Teams receive initial and periodic training in AIDS education, personal care, grief reactions, death and dying information and active listening. Understanding the difficulty that comes from disrupting an ongoing helping relationship, Care Team volunteers are asked to make a one-year commitment to their carepartner and carepartner's family. Teams are partnered with persons who are living with HIV/AIDS from within the community, from faith communities and from referrals by AIDS service agencies.

Matches between caregivers and the carepartner start with the carepartner's perceived needs and requests and the team's capabilities. The team leader and carepartner fill out a calendar based on the carepartner's requests for assistance and volunteers' schedules. Volunteers report higher levels of satisfaction because they don't lose control of their time, and carepartners report higher levels of satisfaction from making the decisions regarding what services are requested.

AIM of Kentuckiana Care Teams Program has been developed to act as a resource to congregations, allowing them to develop or enhance programs of trained and supported volunteer caregivers who provide assistance, encouragement, AIDS education and referral services to people whose circumstances leave them with unmet needs. Congregations already having established helping ministries will find the Care Team's model a beneficial one that can be adapted easily to enhance the ongoing helping responses of the church. This program also provides a network within which congregations can work together more effectively. It serves to strengthen the links between informal caregivers provided by congregations and formal service agencies.

Orphan Care

The growing number of orphans will continue to have a profound impact on the societies in which they live. Orphans may suffer the loss of their entire families, depression, increased malnutrition, lack of immunizations or health care, increased demands of labor, lack of schooling, loss of inheritance, forced migration, crime and exposure to HIV infections.

With orphans comprising up to one-third of the population under age 15 in many countries, it is vital that programs are planned for them that provide long-term care, including family structures and education. The threat to the prospects for economic growth and development in the most seriously affected areas is considerable.

In this section strategies for an immediate crisis-care plan and a long-term plan based on foster parenting are examined. The ultimate goal always should be, where possible, to place children in family-oriented structures.

Crisis Nursery

When we think of a baby nursery, we think of babies freshly washed and powdered, warm and snug in cute bassinets. With tummies full, bottoms dry and surrounded with "TLC" (tender, loving care), they are the picture of contentment. Most parents can't wait for the first opportunity to hold and cuddle their infant.

Orphaned infants in Zambia, however, where HIV/AIDS may infect as much as 25 percent of the population, are not snug in their beds but in critical danger. Jenny Woods, president of Alliance for Children Everywhere (ACE) states, "We see children as young as five years trying to survive on the streets. But what happens to those children under five? What happens to the nursing

146

infant? Those babies who are HIV positive and have no one to hold them or love them?"

The vast majority of Zambian families have no money for formula or milk. It the mother is suspected to have died as a result of AIDS, a wetnurse will often refuse the baby for fear of infecting herself. Too often the infants are buried only days after their mothers die, and young children without hope or home wander the streets trying to survive.

To save the babies, ACE developed a strategy for crisis nursery care for the orphaned infants and vulnerable children. A crisis nursery is a "safe home" in a shanty neighborhood where emergency food and medical supplies are available. Each crisis nursery is attached to a local church or ministry in a local community. The crisis nursery is a place where a pastor or neighbor can find help for an infant who has been left behind when the mother dies and there is no one to nurse the baby and no money available to buy milk. It is not an orphanage. As a child's condition stabilizes, placement is arranged into an extended family, adoptive home or foster home.

With a safe home, orphans can live because immediate intervention is possible. A safe home, some infant formula and good plans are often all that are needed to save the lives of these babies.

ACE encourages groups to conduct baby showers in their homes. Friends bring items as they would for any baby: clothes, diapers, toys, children's vitamins and similar supplies.

Foster Care Programs

Through its foster care program, Inima de Copil in Romania proposes to provide loving, family environments for AIDS children currently living in the state hospital. While living in families, children are also integrated into wider community circles. The objectives of this foundation include:

- providing the children with a normal family life, love, support and respect.
- addressing the children's psychological disorders resulting from prolonged hospitalization.

147

- stimulating the development of each child to his or her maximum potential, both physically and psychologically.

Inima de Copil believes that to see a change in the children and to provide them with some hope for the future, they must be removed from the hospital and placed in a normal family environment. Protection and safety are foundational to a child's healthy development. Home always lies at the heart of a safe and happy childhood. In healthy homes, where relationships are based on love and trust, children develop a sense of self-esteem that molds their identity. Children raised in an institution, many from birth, are denied the blessings of home.

Implementation

In establishing a family placement program, adopting a standard criteria for selecting a foster family is vital. Some families may volunteer strictly for the material benefits that may be offered or other wrong motives. The Department for Child Protection in Galati has the following set of criteria, which are being followed in this project:

1. Status: It is preferable that the partners be legally married and be a stable couple.
2. Condition: The family must have a wholesome, clean residence with a separate room for children, a separate bed for each child, and provisions for sanitation.
3. Provision: The family must have sufficient income to insure adequate provision for the child's needs. Family caregivers must also have good health and be able to work under stressful situations.
4. Aptitude: the parents must show patience, understanding, selflessness, affection, flexibility, understanding of children's needs, and availability to participate in games, care and education of the child.

Foster families are expected to accept and understand the necessity to collaborate with the child's natural family and the social services. They also must carefully consider the needs of their own families and how a sick child may affect the members.

Placing of Children

Once homes are established and families trained, the children can be taken out of institutional care. Removing children from the hospitals can take between twelve to eighteen months. The first step is to contact their natural families (including extended family members). Perhaps if the birth parents can be empowered materially and emotionally to care for their children, it may be possible to place the child back in the home. If this is not possible, then the legal guardianship of a child can be transferred. Since many parents have already signed abandonment statements, relinquishing all responsibility for their children, new patients can sometimes be filtered directly into trained families.

Criteria should also be established for the order in which children will be chosen for placement. These could include age, health, length of living in an institution, and other special needs. Such criteria will enable those involved to choose objectively, not falling into the trap of leaving the ones who are least loved to the last.

Intermediate Step

With two difficulties—finding enough foster families and removing the children from the hospital as soon as possible—an intermediate phase has been implemented. This involves establishing family-type homes where the children can live in groups of four or five. People are hired to work at these homes, and the children are integrated into life in the community. These homes will also be places children can return to if their foster families can no longer care for them.

This step has advantages and disadvantages. It removes the children from the hospital much sooner, but it also creates attachments that will need to be broken if the child is fostered. It also requires more planning and provisions.

Adjusting to Home Life

Both children and their families need to be prepared for the move beforehand. Children should be told about their new family and have time to meet them before removal from the hospital. The parents will need to receive information on the child: family status, institutional history, medical history; behavior difficulties; fears,

149

skills, achievements and interests; name by which he/she likes to be called, preference of toys and hobbies.

Once settled in the home, the children can be placed in some form of schooling, clinic visits arranged and rules for family membership established. The goal is to let the child live as normal a life as possible.

Support Groups

Support groups for foster families are important. Foster parents need access to a weekly meeting where they can express their own fears and problems in a safe environment, share experiences and learn from one another and share resources.

Support groups of children taken from the hospital are also established so they can maintain the relationships formed while in the hospital. This group is run like a play session, providing the children with a non-threatening environment in which to express themselves. Materials are provided that stimulate the children, and also help them to deal with their hopes and fears. For example, toy medical kits can be a tool to discuss medical issues, thus helping the child understand the way treatment is given. Leaders of support groups must have an understanding of child development as well as health issues relating to HIV.

REFLECTION

One hundred children—all affected by HIV/AIDS—gather on a hillside by a lake in Minnesota for a candlelight vigil. The sky darkens. Counselors and parents silently encircle the children and hand each one a small candle secured to a paper plate. The children make their wishes for the future.

This simple candlelight service is poignant. Both celebratory and sad, the candlelight service is often the time when the innermost thoughts and feelings of the children are revealed—when memories of friends or family, now gone, drift along the quiet lake atop 100 small candles floating on paper plates. Where tears flow freely for all the sadness. For all the loneliness. For all the injustice. Yet high above the hillside, hope twinkles in the evening sky.[7]

Hope—what a power-laden word! Hope is the fire we must kindle in the hearts of children overcome with grief and fear through the losses and discrimination caused by HIV/AIDS. This monster threatens to rob them of all they hold most dear: family, home, friends, familiar surroundings, community, education, fun, a normal childhood. Hope, expressed through compassionate care, is the choicest gift our strategies can bestow on children deeply affected by HIV/AIDS.

Notes

1. Susan Hunter and John Williamson, *Children on the Brink,* United States Agency for International Development (no date given), 15.

2. J. A. Colling, *Children Living in a World with AIDS: Guidelines for Children's Participation in HIV/AIDS Programmes* (Switzerland: UNAIDS, 1998), 5.

3. "AIDS at a Glance," *SIMNOW* 88 (Fall 1999), 6.

4. National Council of Children (NCC), *Equity and Vulnerability: A Situational Analysis* (1994).

5. Hunter and Williamson, *Children on the Brink*, 22.

6. Geoff Forster, "Today's Children–Challenges to Child Health Promotion in Countries with Severe AIDS Epidemics," unpublished paper, 1–5.

7. For the Camp Heartland story, see <www.campheartland.com/overview/overview.html>. This reflection is adapted from the account of the candlelight vigil at that website.

11

Facilitating Fun and Learning: Community Education

Glen Slabber

Community education is an important tool to help people express the care and compassion they have in their hearts, feelings that often remain locked up as a result of lack of knowledge. Community education is one way to empower people to look at the problems around them with fresh eyes and to find solutions to those problems in ways that suit their communities and cultures.

Few developing countries have the resources to care for the millions of children who have been and will be orphaned through AIDS in the coming few years. In South Africa, the richest of the sub-Saharan countries, the AIDS pandemic has spiraled out of economic control. The South African government can do no more than offer token medical care to those already living with the disease. The prospect of having to cope with the 1.5 million to 2 million AIDS orphans anticipated by 2005 is beyond the capacity of the South African Social Services and Health Departments. This is typical of most developing countries in Africa and many in Asia, where AIDS is now beginning to spread with frightening speed.

It is against this background that the need to mobilize communities to care for the people living with AIDS in their midst, and the thousands of orphans who will be left, is taking on an ever more urgent aspect. If we are to mobilize communities, we need to educate and empower them. This means educating and empowering the adults.

ADULT LEARNING THEORY AND TEACHING TECHNIQUES

First, we need to realize that adults already have a wide experience of life and a good understanding of the culture and needs of their communities. It is this experience and understanding that we should bring out and use to lead communities to solve the problems they face.

In this respect we are not teachers but rather facilitators who help communities develop their own answers to their problems. The facilitator is as involved in the learning process as those being trained. The only difference between a facilitator and other trainees is that the facilitator has the task of drawing out of the others their knowledge and experience, and helping them channel this into practical solutions.

Being a facilitator can be unpredictable and fun. Questions and reactions are sometimes totally unexpected and refreshing (as well as occasionally leaving us quite nonplussed and searching for a new way of illustrating the point). Still, every contribution by the trainees must be taken seriously. We should never shrug off a contribution as unimportant and never laugh at a trainee. Adults have a strong sense of personal dignity; an unguarded laugh at an answer or a casual dismissal of a comment can stifle discussion and stunt participation.

Good facilitators will be respected by the communities served. At all times we should be courteous and take the trouble to acquaint ourselves with community leaders, maintaining good relationships with them. How we are regarded by the community in which we work will determine how effective we are as educators.

Good communication skills are important. This may sound obvious, but we will often be passing on information that is completely new to those we train and sometimes it will be quite technical in its detail. We need to keep language simple and make sure the translator or local facilitator understands the need for simplicity. Avoid jargon and technical terms as far as possible.

Remember that half the skill of communicating is listening. To listen carefully to the opinions the participants express and the questions they ask encourages them to feel at ease. Careful listening

153

will also help us to understand better the problems and issues with which we need to deal.

The aim of each lesson is to stimulate discussion that leads to action by the trainees. Trainees may have a multitude of ideas about how to care for orphaned children in their community, but if those ideas are not practical or only remain points of discussion, they will be of no use to either the orphans or the community. Aim for practical solutions.

Adults learn quickly about the things that are useful to them. It is therefore important that we encourage participants to talk about the problems they face and then help the whole class to seek a workable solution. The emphasis in a class should be on interaction and discussion with as much participation as possible. We should always be on the alert for constructive feedback.

Remember that when we leave, it is the trainees who will be left to cope with the situation. It is vital, therefore, that the solutions that come out through interaction and discussion be solutions with which the trainees are comfortable. It is tempting to impose on a community a solution that we think is suitable. But without a deep understanding of the culture and the web of relationships within that community, our imposed solution (so clear and logical in our minds) is likely at worst to fail or at best to limp along lamely. The solution that is arrived at must be sustainable once we have gone. Every community is different, with different problems and different ways of solving them.

Many foreign-aid donors have fallen into the trap of assuming they have *the* answer to a community's problems. The story of community education is littered with well-intentioned schemes that have collapsed once the donor has left. There are the ruins of an agricultural scheme in the North West of Zambia that was set up with the intention of teaching the local subsistence farmers to broaden their range of crops (they mostly grow maize). The intention was to teach them about irrigation and about growing fruit trees and a wider range of vegetables to improve their standards of nutrition. Boreholes were sunk; classrooms, student accommodation and research facilities were built. But when the donor left, the center went into a gradual decline despite the best efforts of local staff to keep it going.

154

Why did it decline? Perhaps it was a combination of factors. The center was technically excellent, but it was in an area where agriculture is conducted with the minimum of equipment. It was many miles from the nearest center where equipment could be repaired; when a borehole pump or generator broke down, there was no way of repairing it. It seems that insufficient effort was made either (1) to find out what the local farmers really wanted or (2) to show them the benefits of changing their traditional practices. Fruit trees are a long-term project. This area needs crops that can be planted and reaped in a season to feed a family. The market for a wide range of vegetables is limited because the traditional diet is limited. Further, local farmers did not have the time to spend days at the center being taught about things that had only marginal benefit for them. Neither did they have the means to sink boreholes or buy pumps.

Our education programs should result in projects that are relevant and self-sustaining, not dependent on continued donor funding or outside assistance. The community should be the primary source of all that is needed to sustain the work. There is, of course, a role for donors, particularly in providing start-up funding, but communities need to understand and accept that this funding is likely to be gradually withdrawn and eventually they will need to function on their own. They need to feel they own the work they have been trained to do.

There is an adage in adult education:

> What I hear, I forget.
> What I see, I remember.
> What I do, I know.
> What I discover, I use.

Indeed, tests have shown that people remember

> 20 percent of what they hear,
> 40 percent of what they hear and see,
> 80 percent of what they discover for themselves,
> and 90 percent of what they practice.

Every session of adult community education, therefore, should aim to have a practical outcome and to involve the trainees in the

155

process of education by discovery and practice. Participation by the trainees is important, and training sessions should not be allowed to develop into a formal lecture situation. Of course, there are times when there is no option but to lecture, for example, when teaching subjects that may be beyond the experience of the trainees, such as the details of how HIV/AIDS infects and affects the body. People fall asleep easily when one person holds the stage. However, even in this sort of lesson the points we talk about can be underlined by involving the trainees in role plays that illustrate the main points of the lesson.

We need to be sensitive to the culture of the community with which we are working. If we are dealing with HIV/AIDS education, it is inevitable that we are going to have to discuss issues of sexuality. For many communities this is a difficult subject to talk about in public, particularly if the class is made up of men and women or if it is of the same sex but different age groups. A Kenyan stated that if the topic of sex was raised in a meeting at which his parents or other older people from his village were present, he would have to leave. To remain would be offensive both to him and to the older people.

The principles of community education can be summed up thus:

- Keep lessons relevant to the issues and problems perceived by the community.
- Realize that the community must have a desire to learn how to solve the issues and problems.
- Offer lessons that are as practical as possible; people need to see how the things they learn can benefit their community.
- Encourage participation to help maintain interest and the sharing of knowledge.
- Be sensitive to the culture of the community.
- Keep the classes informal.

THE ROLE OF THE FACILITATOR

In community education the facilitator plays a pivotal role. Before a training session begins, the facilitator should spend time with community leaders to assess their training needs and, with them, construct an appropriate course. If possible, we should spend time identifying likely participants and talking with them about how the course can be made to benefit them and the community.

The course needs to be planned well. A suitable building or site for the course needs to be identified. In many rural areas electricity sources are nonexistent or at least sporadic, so we cannot rely on sophisticated training aids such as videos or overhead projectors; we should use simple materials such as flip charts, chalkboards and blank newsprint. If we are training those in the community who will then go out to train others (and training trainers is a very effective way of spreading community education), then we need to use material and equipment that are readily available locally.

If we are not completely fluent in the local language, then a trustworthy translator is necessary. Better still, we can train a local person to be the facilitator. We then attend as an observer who is simply there as a resource.

In planning a course it is essential to be clear about what the community needs and wants to achieve. This helps keep the lesson plans focused on the right objectives.

Who will be trained? Young people? Older people? Men? Women? A mix of sexes and age groups? The answers will mold the way in which we present the course and its content. We need to fit the timing of the course into the needs of the community rather than expect the community to fit in with a schedule that suits us. If they feel they should be doing other things, they will either drop out of the course or be distracted by their neglected responsibilities—or never attend to begin with.

For instance, if we are teaching women in a rural area, we may need to allow for the fact that a large part of their day must be spent in collecting water and firewood, cooking and looking after children. At a recent course I organized in a rural area of South Africa, the women who attended the course had to get up even earlier than usual to see to their families and then walk several miles to get to the course venue. After the day's lessons they had to walk home, see to the family needs again, and then went to bed later than usual. A five-day, mornings-only course was as much as they could cope with.

Certain times of the year, such as planting and harvest, are particularly busy for rural people. Christmas and Easter are often times when those who live in towns are away visiting their families in their home villages.

Details are important in planning a course or workshop:

- Who will be attending?
- What is the aim of the activity?
- Do we know the training needs of the participants? If not, how can we find out?
- Where is the activity to be held?
- When is the activity to be held?
- How many will attend? (a rough guide for a class or workshop is between 12 and 25).
- What equipment do we need?
- What resources do we have in terms of money, teaching materials, facilitators, and so forth?
- What transport and accommodation arrangements need to be made for facilitators and/or participants?
- What are the arrangements for meals and refreshment breaks?
- Have we included all relevant facilitators and community leaders in the planning?

TEACHING METHODS

There is a wide range of methods we can use. The following list, given in no particular order, details some of the more widely used ones.

Bible Studies

Bible studies are an essential part of any Christian education course. Bible studies can be used as separate lessons in which we show the practical application of God's Word to the skills we are teaching, or they can also be woven into lessons to illustrate particular points we want to emphasize. I think it is important that we seek not only to teach practical skills, but also, as Christians, to build people up in godly knowledge and equip them to share their knowledge of the Lord Jesus Christ with those to whom they minister. As we develop their skills of practical caring and

158

compassion, those skills can build a bridge of good relationships across which the good news of salvation can travel.

Too often we look at the task that faces us as simply a job to be done; how much better to look at the task as a gospel to be preached. For the Christian educator, biblical truths and values should be the bedrock on which the course is built.

Media Aids

Visual aids include pictures, chalkboards, flip charts, videos and slides (where appropriate resources exist), charts, graphs, flannel boards, and so on. These aids encourage participants to discuss the subject and underline the specific points the facilitator wants to bring to the class's attention. Visual aids are of particular importance getting across complex principles that may be new to the participants. They also sum up sessions clearly and quickly. Visual aids are an essential part of most sessions.

Audio aids include tapes, songs and storytelling. In addition to passing on knowledge, a brief audio session is a useful discussion starter. Tapes are also good for distance learning, helping participants prepare at home for a forthcoming session in the class.

Role Plays and Dramas

Role plays and dramas in which the participants devise a real-life situation and act out the parts can be particularly effective in driving a lesson home. For instance, a role play showing a counseling situation will assist people to understand the problems that arise in counseling. Similarly, as participants play other roles, such as the role of someone affected or infected by HIV/AIDS, they gain a better understanding of the feelings and situations of those they are seeking to help. When devising a role play, participants should work out their own story; we need to ensure that, as far as possible, the story reflects a real-life situation.

Many people in developing communities are natural actors and storytellers; to put them into scripted roles may inhibit their gifts of self-expression. This was illustrated particularly well during a role play situation at a Zambian school. A young teacher from England, doing a short spell of teaching in Zambia, wanted her pupils to present a play showing the effects of AIDS on the life of

159

a young man. She carefully scripted the story, making her pupils learn and rehearse their parts until they were word perfect. The children then presented the play to their peers. They were so well drilled that all spontaneity was lost. They performed their parts like robots, marching about the stage and barking out their lines in shrill monotones.

Contrast their performance with a role play we saw later that day. A Zambian teacher wanted to present a similar story. He chose a few pupils, outlined the story to them and sent them away to decide what roles each would play. In ten minutes they returned and gave a fifteen-minute drama that had the members of the audience splitting their sides with laughter. They still drove home the points they wanted to illustrate. The teacher wrapped it all up by briefly summarizing the lesson. It was both memorable and entertaining.

Stories

Illustrative stories bring to life principles and situations and help trainees understand how and why certain situations develop. As they understand better, they can discern similar situations in their communities and explore ways to deal with them.

A typical story might tell of a young mother's struggle to bring up a new baby in her home village when her husband is away in the city looking for work. Factors such as the husband's failure to send money home to support his family, the long distance from a clinic, unfriendly and impatient nurses, drought, the pressing needs of other children and the mother's ignorance of basic health care can all be woven into the story, which ends with the death of the baby. The story is told, and then the trainees analyze the causes of the baby's death. During the analysis the facilitator plays the part of an interrogator asking the trainees why the baby died. They supply the answers, such as "Because the father failed to send money." The facilitator responds to each answer by asking, "But why?" The session goes on until the role of everyone in the story has been discussed and each person's part in contributing to the baby's death is understood. This deeper understanding not only helps participants become more aware of difficult situations in their communities but also can help to change attitudes and remove prejudice.

Question-and-answer Sessions

Question-and-answer sessions help participants to deal with topics and areas of the lessons they might still be uncertain about. They also help achieve openness when discussing culturally difficult subjects such as HIV/AIDS and sexuality.

Personal Experience

Personal experience of another situation is closely allied to drama and role play, but it is specifically designed to allow participants to experience, as closely as possible, a difficult or handicapped situation. Thus, participants might understand a little of what a blind person has to contend with if they are blindfolded and have someone lead them about for a while, perhaps even having to eat a meal blindfolded. Being temporarily blind will underline the feeling of desolation that people experience when health and faculties are lost.

After each session participants should be encouraged to analyze their feelings and reactions and, if necessary, deal with any wrong attitudes or prejudices.

Interviews

Interviewing on a one-to-one basis helps people get to know each other and is a useful preliminary to sessions in which we explore the techniques of counseling. Interviewing should have specific aims, such as finding out personal details, problems, or areas of conflict in one another's lives. Properly conducted, interviewing is an excellent way of discussing sensitive issues.

Discussions

There are a number of discussion formats. Some of the ones we may find useful include the following.

Small-group discussions are good for getting the views, opinions and experiences of all members of the class. Small groups (usually no more than five or six people) encourage participation and concentration. These groups are good for analyzing and solving problems.

Buzz groups are similar to small-group discussions except the size of the group is no more than three people (and ideally only

161

two). The idea of a buzz group is to generate ideas quickly without attempting to analyze them deeply, so these sessions are very similar to brainstorming.

Like the small-group sessions, buzz groups encourage maximum participation and build participants' confidence in their ability to speak out in public. It is noticeable that after small-group and buzz-group sessions the level of participation in large-group lessons improves markedly.

Brainstorming can be done in any size group. During these sessions the participants are encouraged to express as many ideas as they can without trying to assess or analyze them. The facilitator notes them and then at a later session presents them for more detailed discussion. These sessions are useful in helping participants break the mold of traditional thinking; they can result in solutions to problems the group may have previously found impossible to deal with.

Panel discussions followed by questions can give the participants a chance to hear and question experts on issues in which they have little or no experience and thus broaden their knowledge. For instance, people who are HIV positive may talk about the problems they have in their family situation and the worries they have about their children's future once they can no longer support them. These sessions can powerfully motivate people to initiate community care programs.

Large-group discussions are useful in getting the views of the whole group on the issues under discussion. These sessions are also an opportunity for small groups and buzz groups to report back to the entire class.

Demonstrations and Practice

Demonstrations may precede practice. Facilitators might demonstrate good counseling skills and contrast them with a demonstration of poor counseling skills; then the participants practice counseling each other.

Practice is an essential part of adult education. It is by practicing that the participants develop the skills to put what they have learned to good use in the communities they serve. Practice also helps people realize how much they have learned and shows up weak areas that need further development. A combination of demonstration and practice helps participants retain what they have learned and prepares them for the proper use of their skills in the community.

Field Trips

Field trips show the participants work related to the topics about which they are learning. Visits to health clinics to learn about the overall HIV/AIDS situation in their area and the growing problems of and with orphans, for example, will help them see the opportunities for ministry in these areas.

Games

Games are often useful ice-breakers when a group of people who do not know each other come together for the first time. A game designed to help people to remember names helps break barriers of reserve and makes people feel more comfortable in one another's presence.

During the course of a lesson a game can also be used to emphasize and illustrate a point that may be difficult for the participants to grasp. For instance, we use a game designed to illustrate how HIV weakens the body's immune system. The idea is simple: one participant represents the body and another four or five represent the immune system, forming a ring around "the body" with arms firmly linked together. A few other participants are then asked to represent various common diseases and to try to break through the protective circle and attack "the body." Of course, they find it virtually impossible to break through the linked arms. We then get a participant to represent HIV and explain that this disease has the power to break the protective links. Once the links are broken, the various other diseases return and have an easy time breaking through the immune ring, attacking "the body" and (symbolically) destroying it.

It is an energetic game, usually played with great gusto and accompanied by hoots of laughter and shouts of encouragement. But more important, it leaves a clear picture in the minds of players and spectators of how HIV works and its deadly consequences.

Whatever the subject matter and whatever the method—keep it simple!

In all of the above methods we should encourage as much participation as possible. This comes in the form of feedback from the participants as they give their views, express opinions and share experiences. Questions from participants show what they are unsure of and which areas need more teaching and explanation.

Every piece of feedback must be taken seriously. There is always the potential for a question or opinion to be brushed aside as unimportant or even laughed at by the other participants. This is particularly true if the facilitator is looking for a particular answer to be given by the class and the opinion expressed seems irrelevant or even foolish. However, every opinion or question is a genuine contribution to the lesson, and if it seems to indicate a misunderstanding we need to uncover that misunderstanding and put it right. It could also show a smart bit of lateral thinking and be moving toward a solution to the problem under discussion in a way we have missed completely. We need to probe to find the motive behind the unusual feedback.

Feedback can become disruptive and argumentative. The facilitator's job is to keep the lesson orderly and moving toward a constructive conclusion. Even though facilitators are more participant than teacher, the class will still look to us as figures of authority when disputes are to be settled.

Some techniques for dealing with feedback include:

- Repeat the question or comment to the whole class, and then either elaborate on the point or ask the participant to expand on the meaning of his or her opinion or question.
- Always be prepared to give credit for good and useful feedback.
- Always show politeness in dealing with opinions and questions and, by example, encourage all participants to show the same degree of courtesy to one another.
- Adults are likely to have very strong opinions that have been formed by their tradition and culture. Respect these opinions and try to find ways in which they can work for good in the project.

- Be alert to body language in a class. Disagreement or the desire to ask a question can often be discerned by facial expression or posture.

Feedback from the participants is important to help us judge the effectiveness of the lessons.

ILLITERACY

Teaching classes where some participants are illiterate requires particular care but can be very rewarding. People who cannot read or write often have strong memories and come from cultures where remembering and repeating spoken stories are part of their tradition.

Make sure that everything is explained verbally. (Using a good translator or local facilitator is particularly important in these lessons if the facilitator is not fluent in the local language.) If using written materials, read the full text aloud and use plenty of repetition. Allow time for the points of a lesson to sink in, and do not try to teach too much in one session. Allow plenty of time for mental refreshment breaks, and keep the teaching day as short as possible.

Feedback is especially important here, as expressing opinions and asking questions are powerful aids to memory.

Role play, games, demonstrations and pictures are important. The visual and the auditory can reinforce each other.

It can help to appoint one of the literate class members as custodian of written hand-outs. Those who are illiterate can then refer to the custodian if they need reminding about what they have learned.

REVIEW, EVALUATION AND FOLLOW-UP

Review, evaluation and follow up are essential parts of any course, but sadly they are often neglected. Review can be done on a daily basis, emphasizing the main points of the lesson. This can be a good opportunity to correct misunderstandings and strengthen weak points of learning. It is often a good idea to write a summary of the lesson's points on newsprint and post it for the duration of the course.

Especially for a one-day-a-week course (sometimes necessary to fit in with the community's agenda) it is essential to review and evaluate the previous week's lesson before beginning new teaching.

Evaluation should also be carried out at the end of the course. It is often done by asking participants to answer questions aimed at determining what they gained from the course and what areas they think might be improved.

Follow-up is a long-term strategy intended to give course organizers a measure of how the lessons are being put into practice. This may involve return visits and talks with the course participants and possibly community leaders. These visits are not to be seen as "snooping around" to see who is doing the work but rather as opportunities to find out why the skills are not being used (if this is the case) and to determine if further courses would help. An accurate assessment of the effectiveness of the course is also an essential step in reporting back to donor organizations.

An important goal of any follow-up is to encourage the class participants who are now working in the community. Stresses on these volunteers can be much greater than we realize, and part of our work should be to give encouragement. Time spent with community leaders and the families of volunteers to explain what the volunteers are accomplishing can increase both community and family support for workers. Further training is also a source of encouragement as the volunteers learn additional skills and information that will help them better care for others. It helps, too, if volunteers feel they are part of a team and that the team members feel a pastoral responsibility toward one another. Try to prevent volunteers from feeling isolated.

Perhaps a simple uniform and badge will help community workers gain some form of recognition in the community. Recognition is important for their emotional well-being.

Try to ensure that your volunteers are not overburdened with work and that the work load is shared as evenly as possible. Also, some form of remuneration may be necessary to help participants cover costs they incur in their work.

Community education is more than just giving a few lessons and then leaving the people to put into practice what you have

166

taught. Good community education should involve community facilitators for as long as they are needed. It can and will be hard work. However, as we get to know people, see the communities beginning to cope with problems and grow in confidence, we feel a real sense of achievement.

Lessons that are well planned and well presented can be times of good fellowship and shared fun as facilitators and participants learn together.

PART V

Sustenance for Caregivers

12

Training for Compassionate Caregiving

Mary Reeves

CHRIST OUR EXAMPLE

In the time when Christ walked on earth it was unacceptable to touch lepers or even go near them. The attitude of society to these people was one of rejection. But Jesus responded differently. He had an attitude of compassion, which led him to reach out and touch them (Mark 1:40–42).

Our training of caregivers must be aimed at helping them care as Christ would. Following Christ's example—having his attitude of acceptance in helping those with HIV—is an awesome challenge. Compassionate caregiving is not going to happen simply with a list of do's and don'ts but rather through giving information, adding to their knowledge and increasing their understanding, thereby changing attitudes.

During Jesus' time on earth he reached out not only to the sick and dying but also to their family members. Jesus cared for the father of a sick son (Mark 9:17–22); the father of a dying daughter (Luke 8:41–42); and for the mother whose son died (Luke 7:12–14). Jesus' reaching out and caring for others in the family are examples to follow; we should take time also for the relatives of sick and dying children. As one who is around the child and the family, the caregiver can be the presence of Christ to them: his hands, his feet, sharing his love and care.

ATTITUDES AFFECTING BEHAVIOR

In order to perform an activity, knowledge is essential. Understanding and applying knowledge ultimately affects the way we behave or act. Teaching is giving information, but training is changing a lifestyle. We want to train for compassionate care.

Caregivers come into a situation with attitudes that affect the environment. What a different place it is when people are loving, caring and happy in contrast to one where people are angry, unkind, or sad. Attitudes in themselves are unseen, but they are reflected in actions.

Different areas of information and understanding in caring for children with HIV/AIDS affect the care given by the caregiver. In each of several areas we will consider the knowledge necessary to give compassionate care.

Duty

Why are you caring for the child? The answer will reveal the underlying reason or motive the caregiver has for performing a duty. If it is a "job to be done," the goal will be to complete the task, probably as quickly as possible. If it is "to do good," once the duty is done, the goal is accomplished. But if the purpose is to "love and care for a child," the attitudes toward the child and the duty involved are different. The focus is no longer on the activity but the individual. Such a caregiver wants to see the child's physical needs—food, water and hygiene—met, but also seeks to provide the necessary love for the child to grow and develop. The caregiver wants the child and family to have the best quality of life possible.

It is not the place or the things in the place that allow the caregiver to give excellent care. A child can come from a very wealthy house that is a very unhappy home; conversely, a child from a poor home is not necessarily uncared for or unhappy. It is the people in a home who make it what it is. Standard of care does not necessarily depend on facilities. "The child's real environment is the relationships. If these are what they ought to be, he can withstand almost any physical environment."[1] This is very important for the caregivers to understand.

172

Evaluation: Why is the caregiver doing the job? What are his or her motives?

The Child

How caregivers view children affects the care they give. A doctor was heard to say, "I thought children were there to be told what to do!" His understanding of children meant he was not prepared to treat them as individuals with emotions, cares and concerns.

Children need more than food, hygiene, play and education. Every child needs love, along with security, acceptance, significance, understanding and touch. Love and affection are essential to the well-being of a child. These needs are met by the child's parents or the caregivers whom they grow to love and trust.

Children think, respond, react and behave differently from adults. They must not be treated as adults. In so doing, many assumptions of their understanding can be incorrect, and therefore the care given will be inappropriate. Neither should children be considered babies, for then the caregiver will underestimate their need for information and understanding. Children are all individuals, maturing and developing at different rates and in different stages. With understanding, each one can be cared for appropriately.

Evaluation: Has the caregiver an understanding of children, including their basic needs and stages of development?

Change

Children at home are in a familiar environment: they know the people, and tasks are performed in a familiar way, whether changing a diaper or having a meal. Familiarity gives them confidence and reassurance. One basic emotional need—security—is satisfied. But when the child goes into a new situation—a home or a hospital—basic daily routines can be very different. Changes that adults can accept easily may be difficult for a child. The caregiver needs to perceive what these changes mean for the child.

Being in the hospital, away from home, can be threatening for children. Not only are they separated from those they love and trust, but also they are faced with new surroundings and often unpleasant and difficult procedures to go through.

Evaluation: Does the caregiver understand the impact of change on children?

Past Experiences

Many thoughts go through the minds of children; these thoughts are based on children's perspective, their past experiences and previous words they have "heard" or "not heard." Children taken into a new situation may think they are being left by their parents. They may feel alone or isolated, abandoned or rejected. They may believe they are being punished. These ideas may be true in certain situations. However, allowing children to share their thoughts and feelings can prevent present misunderstandings and possible problems in the future; it also helps the caregiver work through these thoughts and feelings with the children.

Caregivers come to recognize the different responses by different children to a similar situation. For example, a younger child going into the hospital may be afraid of being separated from his or her parents. When the parents try to leave the hospital, the young child may scream or refuse to let them go. In contrast, the older child, who has experienced separation, perhaps by attending school, will have greater fear of the potential pain and discomfort associated with hospitals, such as injections. Such a child may be viewed as refusing to cooperate with procedures or being afraid to go to the hospital. The child's pervious experiences of the world and life will affect his or her perceptions, thoughts and ideas.

Evaluation: Does the caregiver understand the importance of experience in the thoughts, questions or fears of children?

Disease

The child with HIV often has repeated illnesses, minor or severe; some can be treated at home while others require hospital admission. The caregiver must also realize the effects of illness. Children will have fears or anxieties related to the sickness and possible investigation or treatment involved. They may experience

174

pain, an area that may be neglected if the caregiver is not aware of how children show pain. Pain may be obvious, expressed through crying, facial expressions, or words spoken. Or a child may express pain indirectly through a general restlessness or crying for affection. If caregivers are aware, they will be ready to respond and to relieve the pain. This is compassionate care—being aware, being alert and then taking action.

The knowledge or lack of knowledge (the understandings or misconceptions of the disease or HIV infection) is important in the actions of the caregiver toward children. If caregivers do not have adequate and accurate knowledge and understanding, they will have unnecessary fears. For example, a caretaker who doesn't know how the virus is spread can be afraid of catching HIV through touch. Not wanting to touch or hold a child cuts off vital communication given through touch. Caregivers' misunderstandings affect their attitudes and ultimately their behavior.

How caregivers handle the children, what they allow the children to do, where they allow them to go, whom they allow them to see are all affected by the caregivers' understanding of disease and illness. Caregivers need to realize that there are times when children can have a "normal" active life and other times when they will require more support and care. Each child's abilities and needs fluctuate over a period of time. Caregivers need to be sensitive to the child at all times, willing to adapt according to the child's condition.

Evaluation: Does the caregiver have a correct understanding of HIV and illnesses that HIV children can have?

Death

Death cannot be avoided when considering HIV, yet death is often not openly talked about, even among adults. Silence about death is often due to personal fears or doubts about what to say. Individuals who have not come to terms with death will be unable to help others effectively. Caregivers need information to gain an understanding and acceptance of death. Caregivers who are unable to talk about death will find it very difficult to help either children or adults.

A child will have questions about death. A caregiver who is not prepared to answer will ignore or avoid the child's questions. Unanswered questions result in the child forming his or her own interpretation of what is happening. Consequently, the child builds his or her own perception of death. How death is portrayed in the media, another source of a child's information, is possibly wrong and probably frightening.

Evaluation: What is the caregiver's perceptions of death? Does the caregiver have unresolved fears and anxieties over death? Is the caregiver able to talk calmly with children about issues related to death?

Family

Children are part of a family, whether their own or one made up of people with whom they are living. Every part of that family will be touched by a child's illness. Members of the family will all have their own thoughts, emotions, reactions and behavior to a sick or dying child—all these will affect the other family members. The impact on a family is greater for a child with HIV because there often are others who are infected. This means there is the fear of one's own death as well as that of a loved one. It raises questions: How quickly will death come for each one? Which one of the family will experience the loss of a loved one? Will the child lose a parent or will the parent lose a child? For some, this may be their first experience of death of a close relative or of a child, with all the dreams and hopes they had for him or her.

In order to enable caregivers to help other family members, they must understand what may be going on within the family. Only then will they appreciate the difficulties family members are experiencing and desire to help each family member. When a child is sick, the extra care that is required, whether at home or in the hospital, the daily routines, family activities and interpersonal relationships within the family are all affected. The responsibilities and pressures increase, causing tiredness, and tiredness causes irritability.

A variety of emotional responses are invoked, including anxiety, grief, fear, guilt and anger. Many questions arise: What did I do wrong? Will my child get better? Why my child? The varied emotions, questions and tiredness affect behavior. It is this behavior which other children in the family experience—not the underlying anxieties. These children have thoughts and perceptions about the behavior they see, which result in them having different and possibly difficult behavior. The caregiver sees a change in the children's behavior, which affects the caregiver's emotions. Thus a cycle is set up. Another factor is the unpredictability of an individual as the emotions and consequent behaviors fluctuate. This causes uncertainty and confusion for others. For example, parents, who would not normally do so, easily get angry or shout at the behavior of other children.

Interaction occurs among all the family members. An example of this interrelation between emotions and behavior among individuals is seen in relation to discipline. Because the child is ill, standards of discipline are altered. For example, parents may become permissive, allowing the child to do or have whatever he or she wants. Or they may pamper the child, giving extra treats or allowing certain things not previously permitted. Other children become jealous or anxious or more demanding, leading to frustration for the caregiver.

Family members may not know or understand why there are changes, and this causes further difficulties and emotional reactions. Therefore, what started out as good for the child ends up affecting all and causing further problems. A caregiver needs to understand and recognize the interactions within the family.

One important factor to remember is that every child expects and deserves an equal share of his or her parents' love, attention and time. As the sick child becomes the focus, the other children do not get their share. The thoughts, fears and questions going through the minds of these children at such a time depend on their experiences and what they have been told or heard. This dynamic may occur not only when a child is sick but also when a child comes into a family or appears "special" for whatever reason.

Well children will have certain attitudes toward sick children. They may feel guilt, believing they are causing the child's illness or that any time the caregiver spends with them takes time the sick child should have. Remember how easy it is for children to have false guilt. At the same time, children may also resent the sick child because he or she takes the caregiver's attention from them or interferes with their activities. They may not know or understand what is happening, and as a result, they may worry or they may feel the caregiver has rejected or abandoned them.

Evaluation: Does the caregiver recognize the interaction of emotions, thoughts and behavior among family members?

APPLYING THE ATTITUDES

As a result of training, a caregiver should realize that he or she is involved in much more than "doing a task." Caregivers are building trust relationships that lead to a deeper understanding of a child's needs. Welling up from this knowledge is the desire to give compassionate care, showering the children not only with practical care but also meeting their needs for love and acceptance.

Part of that compassionate care also will be developing good communication and rapport with the children. Compassionate listening and wise counseling can help children weather many storms. Communication is both talking and listening, both verbal and nonverbal.

TALKING WITH CHILDREN

A caregiver who only is there only to do a task may say, "I have no time to talk to the children" or "I have an important job and it needs to be finished." If caregivers are there for the children and have a desire to understand them, however, it will affect their way of talking with the children—what is said, how it is said, and even whether to speak at all! Caregivers must remember the child is an individual, needing to know and able to understand on his or her level.

Entering into any unknown situation causes anxiety. If we have some idea of what is going to happen, it is easier to cope with difficult or uncertain situations. For example, when a child goes into the hospital, there are many unknowns. Perhaps a child being taken for his first x-ray is told nothing except, "Come along now." That can be threatening and very frightening. The child wonders, Where am I going? What is going to happen? A caregiver who understands that a child has a limited vocabulary can explain that an x-ray is like getting a picture taken. Thus the child's fears will be alleviated.

The child comes not only with a limited knowledge, but also with past experiences. What children have been told, or comments they may have overheard, will also affect their thoughts. For example, a child may have been told, "If you are naughty, I will take you to the doctor" or "If you don't behave, you will get an injection." The child believes, then, that treatment is a punishment or a rejection. When that child has to go into the hospital, he or she feels afraid or guilty. Being alert to children's past experiences and listening carefully to their talk will help caregivers build vital trust relationships.

Evaluation: Is the caregiver challenged to explain carefully situations affecting the child and his or her treatment for AIDS?

Honesty
Children must be told the truth. Failing to be honest (for example, telling a child that a medical procedure will not hurt, even though you know it will) destroys a trust relationship. Even when a true explanation is given on another occasion (perhaps explaining that the procedure will hurt, but not for too long), the child will still be fearful and untrusting. Children learn from experience who to trust and who not to trust. Another aspect of truth concerns keeping promises. It is better not to make a promise than to break our word.

Evaluation: Is the caregiver challenged to be honest and realistic with the children?

Encouragement
Praise and encouragement are vital factors to remember when talking with children. As children go through difficult situations, a word of encouragement may make the difference between a good day and a bad day. Hearing negative words discourages a child, bringing fear and uncertainty. Reassurance is given not only through

179

words, but also—particularly with the young child—through touch.

Evaluation: Does the caregiver see the value in using encouraging words and affirming touch?

LISTENING

Good communication is a two-way street, both speaking and listening. Children, before they are willing to share, need someone who they feel truly cares for them and loves them. They need to know the person is available, willing and ready to listen. Nonverbal as well as verbal communications must be listened to: touch, eyes, expression, posture and emotions. As the child communicates, a caregiver who listens attentively discovers needs, questions and fears. Discovery of the root causes of the problem and ensuing feelings enables the caregiver to respond appropriately, to be understanding and accepting of what children say. It also enables them to answer openly and honestly. Sometimes communication takes place in silence.

For both aspects of communication, talking and listening, the key is time. Only caregivers who realize the importance of communicating with the child are willing to give time to the task. And only caregivers who take time to listen to the children are prepared to care for their deeper needs.

Evaluation: Does the caregiver understand the importance of two-way communication? Does he or she practice it?

FAMILY COMMUNICATION

Individual family members need to help one another in their re-actions and responses to the situations they confront because of HIV. Families will have many questions and fears. They, too, need people who will listen to them honestly and openly. Thus, caregivers need to sense the importance of communicating with family members to understand their interactions. As the family members understand more about the each other's situations, they will be empowered to go through the crisis more easily and with less fear. Knowledge of one another's thoughts will positively

180

affect attitudes, which in turn affect behavior. Greater understanding minimizes problems and difficulties that can arise from failure to communicate or miscommunication.

A child can easily recognize the emotions and feelings of others. The feelings of the caregivers, therefore, are important to the well-being of the child. Whether the child experiences fear and guilt or trust and acceptance depends on whether the caregiver has a positive or negative attitude toward the child's treatment program, parental support system and the situations confronting the child.

Evaluation: Does the caregiver have positive attitudes toward the situation of the children? Do his or her attitudes generate hope and peace?

SPIRITUAL CARE

Caregivers need to recognize that children can know and love Jesus. They can experience the closeness of Christ's presence and comfort through the difficult times, knowing him as a special friend who is with them in every situation. Chubby, a hemophiliac, died at the age of 11 years after a long battle with AIDS. He stated, "I am not afraid to die and go to heaven. It's the being sick part I don't like. Sometimes when I'm real sick I pray to God and ask for my guardian angel to hold my hand. I know God hears my prayer because then my hand feels warm."[2]

With HIV, the awareness of the end of earthly life opens hearts and minds to God and eternity. Children and their family members facing death are open to receiving the truth and the comfort of God. Caregivers need to be taught how to share the gospel in a meaningful way with all family members. Caregivers also must be taught how to answer the questioning doubts of believers going through the trial of a traumatic situation. Caregivers must also learn how to draw the spiritual strength they need for their tasks.

Evaluation: Does the caregiver understand the spiritual needs of the family members and how to answer their questions along their spiritual journey?

SUMMARY

In training the caregiver, we aim to develop a heart for the child, not just head knowledge. Having a heart for children includes training that affects the person's attitudes and, therefore, the practical care given the child. Compassionate caregiving is care that is for the good of the child emotionally, physically, spiritually, socially and intellectually.

The caregiver will be motivated to pay careful attention to the words spoken, listening, the loving actions and the building up of trust relationships. The caregiver who truly understands the children, including their fears and their illness, will be alert to their questions and communications, always ready to help and encourage.

Caregivers have the challenge of caring for each child as an individual. The time and effort we give will be rewarding for the child, especially when we see the children respond and develop healthily. Through compassionate care, caregivers can see the children mature emotionally in their responses and outlook, work through difficulties and hurts as they face the loss of loved ones and the deterioration of their own health and strength.

Through caregivers' compassionate care, family members can avoid problems created by lack of communication or misunderstanding, thus preventing additional fears and anxieties.

As Christ knew about the individual needs of the leper stemming from his disease, he was able to reach out to him without fear and with love and compassion. With knowledge and understanding, caregivers can be equipped to do likewise for children affected by HIV.

Notes

1. Violet Lopes, *The Child: A Simple Child Study Manual*, 2d ed., European Child Evangelism Fellowship (1988), 7.
2. Elaine Deprince, *"Mommy, You Promised,"* Guideposts (March 1996).

13

Keeping Caregivers' Compassion Alive

Phyllis Kilbourn

Caring for someone with AIDS is physically, emotionally and spiritually challenging. The demands can seem endless, overwhelming and unrelenting. Those paying the price of caring for persons affected by AIDS compose a broad spectrum of caregivers. A caregiver could be a young child looking after orphaned siblings or a sick parent; a mother who not only has to confront her impending death, but also the illness of her baby to whom she has passed on the virus; or a grandparent caring for sick or orphaned grandchildren. In developing countries there are few non-family caregivers. Providing care for child caregivers is as vital as for adult caregivers.

Caring for sick children who in all likelihood will regain their health and grow up to live happy, normal, productive lives can be a positive challenge. Caring for children with a debilitating, chronic illness such as AIDS, which usually terminates in death, can be an enormously stressful experience whether the caregiver is a mother, a sibling, a relative, a friend, or other non-family caregiver.

Few understand the tremendous responsibilities and experiences that accompany caring for the critically ill. This is especially true when a child assumes the caregiving role for a critically ill parent. This new role puts children in new and painful situations. Children fear more than anything else the loss of a parent. The depth of the trauma children experience while watching a parent slowly die before their eyes is beyond estimation.

The fear and pain experienced by the parent triggers floods of emotions that continually threaten to engulf the normal coping strategies of the child. It is simply too overwhelming and too painful.

Children also must understand family members on new terms, redefining their roles and re-planning how they will relate to parents and siblings on a daily basis. AIDS changes people's lives in unpredictable ways, making relationships strained and often in conflict. These changes, however, if properly handled, can also cause deeper bonding and stronger relationships within a family.

Caregivers' stresses and problems are compounded by the reality that most of the time vulnerable children and parents are cared for by vulnerable families and reside in vulnerable communities. The communities hardest hit by HIV/AIDS are already severely disadvantaged, with a high incidence of poverty, poor infrastructure and little or no access to even the most rudimentary services. The conditions are conducive to rapid HIV transmission and communities have few resources for caregivers to tap in to.

LOSING THE COMPASSION: THE PATH TO BURNOUT

Working in a situation that produces such overwhelming emotional stress can eventually lead to burnout. The word *burnout* comes from space-program terminology. It describes what happens to the booster rockets that disengage from space vehicles when their fuel is spent. Once out of fuel, the booster rockets are discarded, rendered totally ineffective. This is a good analogy of what can happen to individuals working in high stress settings, such as those caring for people with HIV/AIDS, especially if they are not provided with adequate emotional and spiritual nurturing.

Burnout from caring for the terminally ill can undermine the models of the compassionate care we are trying to establish for children longing to be touched with love and respect. With burnout we lose our capacity to feel, to be deeply touched by the suffering of others. An overload of stress can erode caregivers' effectiveness.

Recent studies show that AIDS caregivers are at risk for burnout because of the unique issues associated with this disease: the

184

stigma attached to AIDS, contagion anxiety, unpredictable symptoms, greater dependency of the patient on caregivers, the loss of those to whom caregivers have been closely attached, limitations on the health-care services due to lack of funding, and the complexity of legal and ethical issues.

While experiencing AIDS-related stress themselves, caregivers have to handle the issues of grief, loss and burnout of the child's family members who also may be participating in the long-term care of their loved ones. Many times family members, or those who have a close relationship with the children, are the primary caregivers. Watching a loved one slowly die extracts a heavy emotional toll. The emotional pain is exacerbated by inadequate medical care, often including lack of funds to purchase the most basic pain-relief medication.

When a caregiver becomes stressed and burns out, both the caregiver and the patient are affected. A stressed-out caregiver lacks the patience and clear thinking to handle the many distresses and crises of a person suffering from chronic illness. Basic needs of the children can be overlooked and insufficient attention given to their overall welfare. Compassion quickly dissipates. Early intervention to prevent burnout is vital.

UNDERSTANDING STRESS THAT LEADS TO BURNOUT

When caregivers come face to face with the realities of caring for a child or an adult with AIDS, stress is bound to occur. Caregivers who experience chronic stress, or have a stress overload, are at risk of becoming emotionally traumatized. Norman Wright describes stress as "any type of action or situation that places conflicting or heavy demands upon a person. These demands upset the body's equilibrium."[1]

SYMPTOMS OF STRESS

Being alert to the symptoms of stress is the first step in the prevention of burnout. Some of the most frequent stress indicators reported are constant fatigue, frequent illnesses, depression marked by bouts of crying, isolation, carelessness in work habits and addictive behaviors.

SOURCES OF STRESS

Once caregivers are alert to the symptoms of stress, they need to be able to identify the sources of stress. These sources are unique for each caregiver. Several sources are listed below. These, and others, can lead to burnout.

Loss of Supportive Structures

Children who have become caregivers find themselves largely confined to the home. Often they have to drop out of school, play or sports activities and church to be available to care for siblings and ailing parents. This not only eliminates the activities that provided them with supportive structures, but they also lose teachers and classmates with whom they have developed meaningful relationships. The pain and frustration, rather than being shared, are stuffed down.

Parents lose the structures provided by the workplace, community activities and the church. Sometimes they even lose the support of the extended family, as family members are consumed with their own grief and anger over their losses.

Difficult Workload

Caregiving for those with AIDS can be an energy-draining, 24-hour-a-day task. With constant interruption of sleep, caregivers do not receive adequate rest. When a sibling or parent is critically ill, there may not even be time to eat nutritious, balanced meals. A heavy workload takes its toll on a caregiver's physical health. When physical health is impaired, emotional reserves are depleted. Tempers flare easily and resentments build up, further eroding the health and well-being of a caregiver.

Increase in dependency as the illness progresses adds to the workload of already stressed-out caregivers. The amount of dependency shifts with the person's health. Children with AIDS may want to be held more. Adults with AIDS may want the caregiver to be more accessible. Mental impairment may take away whatever independence the sick person has had and greatly increases the need for constant care and observation.

Anger

Injustice is a painful issue to confront, especially when it concerns children who have been infected with HIV/AIDS through prostitution or sexual abuse. Caring for children who have been bereft of parents, siblings and friends through the actions of people who have no concern for the untold sufferings they are inflicting on others can evoke intense rage.

Knowing that God is a just God, who promises to set the record straight one day, gives hope in the darkest situations. And, within the context of God's faithfulness, we can let go of those aspects of the children's lives that are outside our sphere of control yet trouble us deeply.

Caregivers may also begin to feel resentful and angry about constantly having to accommodate the person with AIDS and keep the peace when disagreements arise over care or issues such as confidentiality. However, caregivers are usually reluctant to show their anger to the person in their care, so they find other ways to deal with it. This too often means suppressing it and denying their feelings of pain and anger or venting their anger on other people with whom they have a relationship. If unresolved, this rage continues to boil deep within the caregivers' emotions, rendering them emotionally crippled and certainly drained of compassion. Anger and resentment can also manifest themselves through headaches, ulcers and other pain.

Relationships

A mutual and trusting relationship between a patient and a caregiver lies at the heart of successful caregiving. Yet caregivers of terminally ill patients tend to restrict that relationship, not letting it become too close. When patients become friends, the pain and grief at the time of death is more difficult to handle.

Considering the dynamics of caring for a critically ill person, along with the ramifications of that illness—especially as it becomes a more dependent relationship—caregivers need to consider how to maintain a good relationship. Conflicts of the heart and mind drain precious energy from caregivers.

Relationships between family members and other caregivers also are important to the overall well-being of everyone concerned.

In even the most ideal situations, interpersonal relationship problems erupt. Friction is bound to occur, especially among other family members. Flexibility, tolerance, patience and forgiveness are vital tools for minimizing conflicts in a caring relationship.

Grief and Loss

Grief is a normal and natural response to loss. While caregivers are handling their own issues of grief and loss, they also have to address grief issues, cumulative loss and burnout among many friends and family members who are dealing with the long-term care of loved ones. In trying to act compassionately, it is easy for caregivers to lay aside their own emotional pain. Keeping grief bottled up inside increases a caregiver's pain.

HANDLING STRESS: KEEPING THE COMPASSION ALIVE

Kairos[2] defines caregiving as an art that requires subtle balancing of our needs with our desire to serve others. Burnout happens when we fail to replenish ourselves. Serving others then ceases to be fulfilling, and we are depleted of physical, emotional, and spiritual resources for compassionate care. Reducing stress is a primary goal of prevention.

Caregivers need holistic care to avoid burnout, an approach that looks at emotional, physical, relational and spiritual factors. Caregivers need to think creatively about options such as setting limits on responsibilities, delegating tasks and being properly trained and equipped for the task.

Caregivers also need to learn how to strengthen their inner resources to cope with pressure-filled schedules, death and grieving and unexpected demands. Perhaps most important, they must learn to let go those aspects of life that are beyond their control. They need to evaluate constantly how they can best care for themselves in order to be at their best as effective, compassionate caregivers.

The following are some practical ideas for preventing burnout and keeping the compassion alive.

Maintain an Emotional Balance

When caring for terminally ill children, caregivers need to guard against over-identifying with the children's emotional pain. While

188

we don't want to over-identify with the children's pain to the point where it cripples us emotionally, we also need to watch for the opposite—emotional detachment, allowing the emotional space we keep between a child and ourselves to become a gulf between us. If we become emotionally detached, we shut down because we can no longer cope with the child's issues of loss and grief. Fatigue often accompanies and heightens emotional detachment. Caregivers are just too tired to care. Caregiving then simply becomes a matter of "putting in our time" rather than offering the gift of compassion and love.

Recognize Limitations

Caregivers must frequently reevaluate their task of caregiving, especially to pinpoint the areas of greatest stress. From their findings they can plan to reduce stress by setting limits on their responsibilities and involvements.

It is important to set limits or boundaries for what caregiving includes and does not include in each situation—especially regarding work schedules. No one can effectively care for a person 24 hours a day without breaks. Caregivers need to set limits not only on their time but also on their energy, resources and competencies. To be good stewards of what God has given us, we need to make wise choices regarding our use of resources.

With a little creative planning, other options can be used to reduce stressful situations. Sometimes errands or other time-consuming tasks can be shared, or family members can assume some of the responsibilities that are overloading caregivers.

Take Breaks

Caregivers, especially family members, need to distance themselves from their caregiving burdens daily—even if only for an hour. They need time with a healthy adult for social interaction, a friend they can confide in. Distance can help caregivers keep their perspective—and patience. A break for a mother may simply mean a walk around the neighborhood or meeting a friend for coffee. Group social activities that allow caregivers to detach from their work should be planned frequently. Caregivers need to maintain a healthy sense of humor.

Outlet for Venting Feelings

Sometimes stress results when caregivers cannot vent their feelings of guilt, anger and frustration. Support groups are safe places to express pent-up feelings. Other healthy ways to defuse feelings include:

- taking a walk and enjoying the beauties of nature.
- meeting with a trusted friend for sharing and prayer.
- expressing feelings through music, interpretive dance, drama or role play, journaling and so on.
- learning relaxation techniques.

Personal Care

Caregivers need to attend to their own needs to keep healthy physically and emotionally. This includes maintaining good eating habits, sufficient rest, regular exercise, recreation and free time. Those responsible for caregivers can also help them by providing personal and professional support.

Caregivers must balance their own needs with the needs of others, not letting the needs of others drain them of their energy and vitality. Burnout occurs when we fail to renew our "fuel supply." Caring then ceases to be fulfilling, and we become depleted.

Spiritual Nurture

Nurturing our spiritual lives is one of the most vital things we can do to prevent burnout. Without being connected to an infinite and divine power source, we will inevitably run out of steam. To avoid burnout, we need to watch and guard against spiritual apathy, which usually results from putting our spiritual needs last on our list of priorities. We need to watch for a decline in spiritual disciplines such as personal Bible study, prayer, times of quiet reflection and corporate worship. Failing to fill our spiritual needs not only leads to burnout but also could lead to failure due to sin as a result of our moral boundaries becoming cloudy and undefined.

Support Sessions

When caring for AIDS patients, caregivers desire to give all the compassionate care possible to ease the pain and suffering of those

190

for whom they care. But many conflicting ideas, pressures and situations may cause the caregiver to feel anything but compassionate. If a support group is not provided for caregivers (see next section), then provision must be made for ongoing sessions in which caregivers can express their fears, anger, guilt, frustrations and grief over what they are experiencing. In some situations, sessions apart from the support group may be more satisfactory. The sessions may prepare the caregivers for a more productive time in their support networks.

Support Groups

Caregivers must be provided with supportive networks to cope with the constant loss, pain and grief of children and their families. Caregivers also need those with whom they can share their own personal problems and difficulties in caregiving. It is helpful to have non-caregivers in the group, such as a trusted pastor or friend. Being on the "other side of the problems," they can bring a fresh point of view into the discussions.

Remember, children also need support groups where they can get advice, be trained in proper caregiving, learn how to avoid becoming infected and keep themselves in good health generally. Their support groups need to monitor the children's schedules, making sure they get adequate rest, food and breaks when the pressures of caregiving become too great.

Time together in support groups provides caregivers an opportunity to address any team, patient or family conflict issues along with seeking solutions. It also provides opportunities to encourage those who may be feeling down or isolated, to share areas of expertise along with offering assistance and prayer support when a caregiver feels overwhelmed.

Plan specific, frequent times for caregivers to share together in an emotionally safe environment, a place where they can feel free to vent their anger, frustrations, fears, inadequacies and other feelings or emotions that trouble them. Expressing their feelings allows caregivers to find a renewed perspective on the depth of their emotions and where the source of these reactions lie.

Listening is essential to talking! Support group members must be encouraged to listen with their hearts as well as their ears, allowing others to express their feelings and thoughts. Although honest and open sharing is encouraged, caution must be taken not to push anyone into opening up prematurely. Some people need extra time and space to reflect and work through issues before sharing openly. Assurance of confidentiality also facilitates sharing.

When a warm, caring and nurturing environment is provided for sharing, along with strong prayer support, clarification of issues will occur resulting in new perspectives and a restoration of hope.

TURNING BURNOUT TO BLESSING

To keep the compassion alive, it is vital that caregivers nurture and replenish each aspect of their life: heart, mind, spirit and body.

Times of burnout can become opportunities to reevaluate personal and professional goals, a time to refocus on our God-given calling of helping others. Evaluation forces us to reset our priorities, responsibilities and expectations.

Burnout may begin with depletion, but it can end with an emotional, spiritual and physical renewal that enables us to reclothe ourselves with compassion. Once reclothed, we again can express the compassion of Christ in every detail of our caregiving, adding the "jam" of compassionate care.

Notes

1. H. Norman Wright, *Crisis Counseling* (Ventura, Calif.: Regal Books, 1993), 59.

2. Kairos Support for Caregivers, "Are You ARB+" (San Francisco, Calif.: Kairos).

PART VI

First-Person
Perspective

14

Stefanie's Courageous Journey: A Tribute to Compassionate Caregivers

Phyllis Kilbourn,
with poems by Stefanie Sakuma

Children need courage, tremendous courage, to face the ravaging effects of AIDS. From what reservoir can children draw the courage they so desperately need? Often they are consumed with pain, fear, emotionally drained and physically weak—out of human resources. Can they, too, draw upon spiritual resources to get them through the dark and difficult days? Yes! Especially if they have been blessed with compassionate caregivers who have equipped them with these spiritual resources.

Stefanie Sakuma's parents equipped her with rich spiritual resources. Through God's help, Stefanie was able to comment, "I have never really suffered. I have my family and God who love me." Yes, family or other compassionate caregivers are indeed a major source of strength, especially when their strength is rooted in a loving heavenly Father whose heart longs to wrap each suffering child in his strong and loving arms, bestowing on his beloved children those needed healing touches.

Stefanie, whose story you read in chapter 3, was well acquainted with pain, fatigue, fear, loneliness and despair. But these "foes" did not consume her because her parents, along with the gift of their compassionate care, also gave her the gift of knowing Jesus

195

as her Lord and Savior. Stefanie learned that Jesus could comfort her, calm her fears and give her hope in a future in spite of her situation. She also learned that "joy is not the absence of sorrow, but the presence of the Lord."

Her parents state, "Yes, children are resilient, but I know if it were not for a strength and power beyond ourselves, she could not have bounced back time and time again. From the time that she was 19 months old, when we found out she had hemophilia, God in Jesus Christ has not ceased to walk beside us. At every point of despair—crippled ankles, lupus, infections—he never has failed to be the God of all comfort and sufficiency."

Stefanie found joy and comfort in recording in poetry her experiences as she confronted the challenges of living with AIDS. In her poems she freely expressed her feelings of pain, fear, loneliness and frustration. But she never stopped there! She always went on to record God's loving responses to these times of turmoil and pain; she went on from her times of despair to reflect the hope Jesus always provided.

Stefanie, often on crutches or in a leg cast from joint and ankle bleeds, memorized Psalm 23 at age four and won her first Bible. Both were sources of continual encouragement in her life. The psalm focuses on gifts that all compassionate caregivers can and must bestow on children who otherwise face a bleak future: hope, peace, joy, knowledge of Jesus as one who longs to be present in the midst of their pain and suffering, and a future both in their short stay on earth and for all eternity.

Stefanie will introduce herself through a letter written in her book of poetry. These poems were written between the ages of 9 and 11. The journey for Stefanie was short, yet she walked with courage and faith in the Shepherd she loved and knew so well. Stefanie died from AIDS contracted from a blood transfusion during a treatment for hemophilia.

The following selections from Stefanie's poems, from her book *Walking with My Lord*, are accompanied by verses from Psalm 23.

> *My name is Stefanie Sakuma. I am 11 years old and started writing poems when I was 9.*

I wanted people to share my poems with other people. I thought it could help other people to know God. I know that God has helped me through bleeds [hemophilia], being on crutches, having lupus, many transfusions and through days at the hospital. If I didn't know God, I'd have been ready to give up a long time ago.

Sometimes I wonder if I fear death, but I know I don't because life after death is better than life on earth. The painfulness of my body will be gone. Sometimes I think pain will never end or a bloody nose will never stop. I still have hope in God because He gave me all these handicaps to show other people about Him. Even when I didn't feel like overcoming, He brought people to visit me and to pray for me. He gave me new strength each time.

Reality of God's Presence with Us

The LORD is my shepherd, I shall not want. (Ps 23:1)

Bless the Day
I bless the day
That Jesus came into my heart
This is the day I praise Him
And I know this is just a start.

Now I can share the news
'Cause now I understand
The glory of God is with me
He guides me by His hand.

"When I am afraid, I will put my trust in Thee."
Psalm 56:3

Rest–Quietness of Heart

He makes me lie down in green pastures;
he leads me beside still waters,
   he restores my soul.
He leads me in right paths
   for his name's sake. (Ps 23:2)

Walking with My Lord
I went walking with my Lord
　　By the Galilee.
I went walking with my Lord
　　Just my Lord and me.
And then my Lord
　　He asked me,
"Have you been acting as
　　my messenger?
All the people need to know Me
　　Should an accident occur."

The Garden
Sitting in the garden
I watch the birds and bees
Flying near the flowers
Nesting in the trees.

Sitting in the garden
I watch the jays and quail
Flying round so freely
To all nature hail!

Peace and Comfort

Even though I walk through the darkest valley,
　　I will fear no evil;
for you are with me;
　　your rod and your staff—
　　they comfort me. (Ps 23:4)

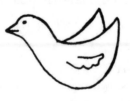

Peace
Peace be with you
Don't tell someone what's wrong or right

Peace be with you
Tell them what's good in God's sight.

Don't tell them something that isn't true
Peace be with you
Tell them something they'll understand.
Peace be with you.

Freedom from Fear

You prepare a table before me
in the presence of my enemies. (Ps 23:5a)

Fear
It happens in the night
When fear comes on me.
There is not a way out of this
As far as I can see.

But then I watch and look
And see the things around me.
The thing I see is an angel,
I know it has to be.

The angel stands to guard me
From all the things I fear
So then I go to sleep
and everything is clear.

Hope

You anoint my head with oil;
my cup overflows. (Ps 23:5b)

Any Power
Is there any power greater
Than that that praises God?
Is there any power greater
Than that that changes Aaron's rod?

Shall we sing of some other god?
That's just another illusion.

> Or shall we ever sing
> Of the rightful Lord,
> God, our King!

Blessings of God

> Surely goodness and mercy shall follow me
> all the days of my life. (Ps 23:6a)

The Lord Is With Me
Lying in a hospital bed
Trying not to despair
But I know the Lord is with me
And so His child I'll be.

I know the Lord is with me
And I'm blessed from all He's done,
So I'll praise Him all the day
Everywhere and in every way.

An Eternal Future

> I shall dwell in the house of the LORD
> my whole life long. (Ps 23:6b)

Glory Place
(Stefanie's last poem)
I'll tell you a story
Of a place where of all glory
A place where rivers run,
A place beyond the sun,
A place after death,
After a life of struggles and strife.
And no one knows where it lies;
It's a place where no one dies;
It's a place where God is alive.

Stefanie would want her words of comfort, hope and life to bless suffering children everywhere. Stefanie dreamed of becoming a missionary-doctor, healing people while spreading the Christian gospel. Even though these aspirations were cut short, caregivers can help fulfill her dream by passing on the blessings she received as gifts to other suffering children through compassionate care.

Her parents add a plea for the church "to open its heart and arms as a place of refuge and support to the chronically and terminally ill in demonstration of God's love." What an awesome privilege—and responsibility!

Appendix:
Resources for Ministry
and Networking

Books

Arnold, Lynda. *My Mommy Has Aids*. Blue Bell, Pa.: Dream Publishing, 1998.

Bartlett, John G., M.D., and Ann K. Finkbeiner. *The Guide to Living with HIV Infections: Developed at the Johns Hopkins AIDS Clinic.* 3d ed. Baltimore, Md.: Johns Hopkins University Press, 1996.

Brenner, Avis. *Helping Children Cope with Stress.* San Francisco: Jossey Bass, 1984.

Coles, Robert. *Be a Friend: Children with HIV Speak.* Morton Grove, Ill.: Albert Whitman & Company, 1994.

Corr, C., and D. Corr, eds. *Handbook of Childhood Death and Bereavement.*

New York: Springer Publishing Company, 1996.

Dane, Barbara, and Carol Levine, eds. *Aids and the New Orphans: Coping with Death.* Westport, Conn.: Auburn House, 1994.

Farmer, Paul, ed. *Women, Poverty and AIDS.* Monroe, Me.: Common Courage Press, 1997.

Geballe, Shelley, and Warren Andiman, eds. *Forgotten Children of the Aids Epidemic.* New Haven, Conn.: York University Press, 1995.

Hoffman, Patricia L. *AIDS and the Sleeping Church: A Journal.* Grand Rapids, Mich.: Eerdmans, 1995.

Hunter, Susan, and John Williamson. *Children on the Brink: Strategies to Support Children Isolated by HIV/AIDS.* Washington, D.C.: USAID, 2000.

Jurkovic, Gregory J. *Lost Childhoods: The Plight of the Parentified Child.* Bristol, Pa.: Brunner/Mazel Publishers, 1997.

Lester, Andrew D., ed. *When Children Suffer: A Sourcebook for Ministry with Children in Crisis*. Philadelphia: The Westminster Press, 1987.

Monahan, Cynthia. *Children and Trauma: A Parent's Guide to Helping Children Heal*. New York: Lexington Books, 1993.

Nouwen, Henri J. M., Donald P. McNeill and Douglas A. Morrison. *Compassion: A Reflection on the Christian Life*. New York: Image Books Doubleday, 1982.

Shelp, Earl E., and Ronald H. Sunderland. *AIDS and the Church: The Second Decade*. Louisville, Ky.: Westminster/John Knox Press, 1992.

Sweeney, Daniel. *Counseling Children Through the World of Play*. Wheaton, Ill.: Tyndale House Publishers, 1997.

Webb, N. B., ed. *Helping Bereaved Children*. New York: Guilford, 1993.

TALC

Strategies for Hope is a Teaching Aids at Low Cost (TALC) project founded by ActionAid to promote informed, positive thinking and practical action for coping with AIDS in developing countries. Its series of book/booklets includes:

> *Open Secret: People Facing up to HIV and AIDS in Uganda*
> *Living Positively with AIDS: The AIDS Support Organisation (TASO), Uganda*
> *AIDS Management: An Integrated Approach*
> *Meeting AIDS with Compassion: AIDS Care and Prevention in Ghana*
> *AIDS Orphans: A Community Perspective from Tanzania*
> *The Caring Community: Coping with AIDS in Urban Uganda*
> *All Against AIDS: The Copperbelt Health Education Project, Zambia.*

Other titles in the series focus on Zimbabwe, Côte d'Ivoire, India and Kenya.

ALSO available from TALC are several videos, including:

> *Under the Mupundu Tree,* which describes a home-care program in Zambia.
> *The Orphan Generation,* community-based care and support for children with AIDS.

HIV/AIDS Counselling: The Taso Experience, counseling, care
and support for people with HIV/AIDS.
Open Secret, which details people facing up to HIV and
AIDS in Uganda.

TALC booklets and videos can be ordered in Europe from
TALC on line at s0tratshope@aol.com, or in the U.S.A. by e-mail
to books@pactpub.com. At TALC's website, www.stratshope.org
one can also order a catalog and/or ask to be put on TALC's
mailing list.

Internet Books, Information and Resources

For background information and resources about children and
AIDS, see websites of organizations such as The AIDS-HIV Resource Center, World Bank, Childhope USA, Captive Daughters,
World Congress Against Commercial Exploitation of Children,
UNAIDS, ActionAid and the Children with AIDS Project, and topics such as "Children's Health and Human Rights," "AIDS as a
Development Issue," and "The Rights of the Child in the Context
of HIV/AIDS." Many resources can be located by entering com-
binations of key words such as *children, AIDS, rights, resources,
development,* and so forth in an Internet search engine.

Resource Groups

Regional AIDS Interfaith Network (RAIN) is a ministry encouraging people of all faiths to respond compassionately to persons
with HIV/AIDS through education and the development of Care
Teams to enhance the quality of life for persons affected by AIDS.
Its publication is *Raindrops.* Check its website for the regional of-
fice in your area.

KARIOS is a family support network and a special outreach
program that provides on-site training to staff of hospitals and
agencies. A 14-minute video, "Together We Care," discusses a
variety of issues caregivers confront and the importance of support. The video and other caregiver tools can be obtained from
KAIROS, 114 Douglass Street, San Francisco, CA 94114 (or call
415-861-0877).

He Intends Victory (HIV): A Christian Ministry to Those Affected by AIDS was established to lead the body of Christ toward a compassionate, balanced, informed ministry to the HIV/AIDS community. Contact person is its president, Rev. Bruce Sonnenberg, PO Box 18499, Irvine, CA 92623 (1-800-HIV-HOPE or fax 714-474-0610).

Faith, Hope and Love Community Services, Inc. (FHL) is committed to providing HIV testing, early intervention programs, pediatric respite, HIV/AIDS training and other services to anyone affected or infected by HIV/AIDS. Its address is PO Box 10471, Colorado Springs, CO 80932-0471 (719-596-0072).

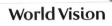

Children and Mission

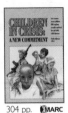

CHILDREN IN CRISIS
Phyllis Kilbourn, editor

AIDS, abandonment, sexual abuse, forced labor, war, urban violence and girl-child discrimination destroy far too many children's lives around the world. Kilbourn moves you to a biblical response to these global crises.

304 pp. MARC
1996
R-016
$21.95

SEXUALLY EXPLOITED CHILDREN
Working to Protect and Heal
Phyllis Kilbourn and Marjorie McDermid, editors

A practical, hands-on tool for those who want to respond to the needs of hurting children who have been exploited by the sex industry.

248 pp. MARC
1998
K-009
$24.95

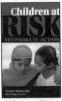

HEALING THE CHILDREN OF WAR
Phyllis Kilbourn, editor

Children are the most innocent and helpless victims of war. The increasing number of children who are victims of war is startling. This handbook is for those who are ready to minister to children who have suffered deep traumas.

330 pp. MARC
1995
R-007
$21.95

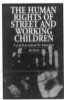

STREET CHILDREN
Phyllis Kilbourn, editor

Kilbourn orients workers among street children and explains who street children are, where they can be found and why they are on the streets. She also gives practical advice for ministering to homeless children.

330 pp. MARC
1997
K-008
$23.95

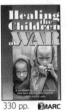

CHILDREN AT RISK
Networks in Action
Patrick McDonald with Emma Garrow

This is the powerful story of building the Viva Network, a strategic response to at-risk children. McDonald provides practical suggestions enabling Christians to mobilize their resources and offer a better future to the world's children.

152 pp. MARC
2000
K-012
$12.95

HUMAN RIGHTS OF STREET AND WORKING CHILDREN
A Practical Manual for Advocates
Iain Byrne

This volume is a one-stop guide for experienced field advocates or non-specialists and explains how to use regional and international treaties and mechanisms to protect and defend street and working children when national law fails.

278 pp.
1998
Y-011
$47.50

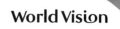

Holistic Mission

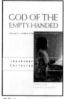

GOD OF THE EMPTY-HANDED
Poverty, Power and the Kingdom of God
Jayakumar Christian
The author explores the relationship of poverty to powerlessness by masterfully integrating anthropology, sociology, politics and theology. Avoiding easy answers, he offers a new paradigm that can shape our responses to the poor and provide a workable framework for grassroots practitioners.

224 pp. **MARC**
1999
Y-003
$21.95

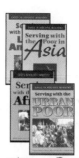

SERVING WITH THE POOR SERIES
various authors
Case studies in holistic ministry challenge commonly accepted theories with the reality of mission from a grassroots perspective. this series presents valuable, practical lessons that have shaped and influenced mission initiatives.

various **MARC**
$12.95-16.95

HOLISM IN DEVELOPMENT
An African Perspective on Empowering Communities
Deborah Ajulu
Does God's bounty belong to all God's children? Dr. Deborah Ajulu, a new and important African evangelical voice, explores how biblical ethics apply to the escalating challenges presented by entrenched poverty in communities around the globe.

224 pp. **MARC**
2001
Y-019
$22.95

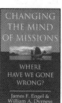

CHANGING THE MIND OF MISSIONS
Where Have We Gone Wrong?
James F. Engel and William A. Dyrness
The world is rapidly changing, but is mission? The new millennium has arrived, bringing even greater global and cultural changes. Yet, according to the authors, missions has remained the same. Here they offer a courageous analysis of the challenges facing Western missions and point the way forward.

189 pp.
2000
S-069
$12.95

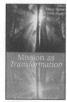

MISSION AS TRANSFORMATION
A Theology of the Whole Gospel
Vinay Samuel & Chris Sugden, editors
Holistic mission integrates proclamation, evangelism, church planting and social transformation in a seamless whole of Christian mission. This volume traces the development of holistic mission, provides the biblical and theological foundations for it and explores its practical expressions.

522 pp.
2000
M-067
$24.95

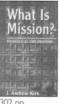

WHAT IS MISSION?
Theological Explorations
J. Andrew Kirk
What does "mission" mean today? How can we "make disciples of all nations?" Kirk addresses these important questions as he strips mission of its old associations with colonialism and looks anew at the underlying theology of mission. He reminds us that our task is God's mission.

302 pp.
2000
T-003
$19.95

MARC

1-800-777-7752 • www.marcpublications.com
marcpubs@wvi.org • 626-301-7789 fax

World Vision

Relief, Development and NGOs

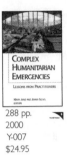

COMPLEX HUMANITARIAN EMERGENCIES
Lessons from Practitioners
Mark Janz & Joann Slead, editors
In this volume, experienced practitioners address the question of how we can respond appropriately to CHEs by linking conceptual and theoretical thinking to practical application at the grassroots level.

288 pp.
2000
Y-007
$24.95

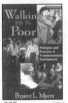

WALKING WITH THE POOR
Principles and Practices of Transformational Development
Bryant L. Myers
Drawing on theological and biblical resources, secular development theory and work done by Christians among the poor, Myers develops a theoretical framework for transformational development and provides cutting-edge tools for those working alongside the poor.

288 pp.
1999
Y-008
$21.95

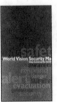

WORLD VISION SECURITY MANUAL
Safety Awareness for Aid Workers
Charles Rogers and Brian Sytsma, editors
Global trends and recent events signal the growing vulnerability of international aid workers and missionaries. Filling the void for safety manuals, this pocket-sized book is designed to help create a complete personnel safety policy.

148 pp.
2000
S-022
$14.95

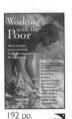

WORKING WITH THE POOR
New Insights and Learnings from Development Practitioners
Bryant L. Myers, editor
Here, development practitioners from around the world struggle to overcome the Western assumption that the physical and spiritual realms are separate and distinct from one another in answering the question, How do Christian practitioners express authentically holistic transformational development?

192 pp.
1999
Y-002
$16.95

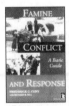

FAMINE, CONFLICT AND RESPONSE
A Basic Guide
Frederick C. Cuny
Cuny was a highly respected disaster relief practitioner and strategist. Before he disappeared in Chechnya in 1995 he completed this important book on famine. In it, he proposes immediate and lasting solutions to famine by identifying its underlying causes and focusing on livelihood, not just survival.

174 pp.
1999
Y-004
$23.95

DO NO HARM
How Aid Can Support Peace—or War
Mary B. Anderson
When international assistance is given in the context of violent conflict, the aid can either help reduce tensions or prolong the fighting. This book helps aid agencies and practitioners know how to provide humanitarian aid and support peace.

160 pp.
1999
F-023
$16.95

MARC

1-800-777-7752 • www.marcpublications.com
marcpubs@wvi.org • 626-301-7789 fax